Embryology Workbook

Embryology Workbook

Preeti Sonje
MBBS, MD (Anatomy)

Professor
Department of Anatomy
Dr DY Patil Medical College Hospital and
Research Centre, Pimpri, Pune

Neelesh Kanasker
MBBS, MD (Anatomy)

Associate Professor
Department of Anatomy
Dr DY Patil Medical College Hospital and
Research Centre, Pimpri, Pune

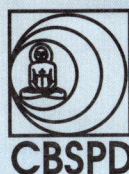

CBSPD

CBS Publishers & Distributors Pvt Ltd

New Delhi • Bengaluru • Chennai • Kochi • Kolkata • Lucknow • Mumbai
Hyderabad • Jharkhand • Nagpur • Patna • Pune • Uttarakhand

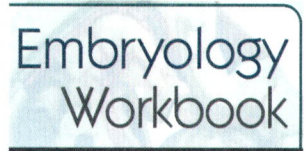

ISBN: 978-93-90046-00-3

First Edition: 2020
Reprint: 2021, 2023

Published by Satish Kumar Jain and Produced by Varun Jain for

CBS Publishers & Distributors Pvt Ltd

4819/XI Prahlad Street, 24 Ansari Road, Daryaganj, New Delhi 110 002, India.
Ph: 011-23289259, 23266861

Website: www.cbspd.com
e-mail: delhi@cbspd.com

Corporate Office: 204 FIE, Industrial Area, Patparganj, Delhi 110 092
Ph: 011-4934 4934   Fax: 011-4934 4935   e-mail: publishing@cbspd.com; publicity@cbspd.com

Branches

• **Bengaluru:** Seema House 2975, 17th Cross, KR Road, Banasankari 2nd Stage, Bengaluru 560 070, Karnataka, India
  Ph: +91-80-26771678/79   Fax: +91-80-26771680   e-mail: bangalore@cbspd.com
• **Chennai:** 7, Subbaraya Street, Shenoy Nagar, Chennai 600 030, Tamil Nadu, India
  Ph: +91-44-26680620, 26681266   Fax: +91-44-42032115   e-mail: chennai@cbspd.com
• **Kochi:** 42/1325, 1326, Power House Road, Opp KSEB, Power House, Ernakulum Kochi 682 018, Kerala, India
  Ph: +91-484-4059061-65,67   Fax: +91-484-4059065   e-mail: kochi@cbspd.com
• **Kolkata:** 147, Hind Ceramics Compound, 1st Floor, Nilgunj Road, Belghoria, Kolkata-700056, West Bengal, India
  Ph: +033-25633055, 033-25633056   e-mail: kolkata@cbspd.com
• **Lucknow:** Basement, Khushnuma Complex, 7 Meerabai Marg (Behind Jawahar Bhawan),Lucknow-226001, UP, India
  Ph: +91-522-4000032   e-mail: tiwari.lucknow@cbspd.com
• **Mumbai:** PWD Shed, Gala no 25/26, Ramchandra Bhatt Marg, Next to JJ Hospital Gate no. 2, Opp. Union Bank of India, Noorbaug, Mumbai-400009, Maharashtra, India
  Ph: 022-66661880/89   e-mail: mumbai@cbspd.com

Representatives

• Hyderabad	0-9885175004	• Jharkhand	0-9811541605	• Nagpur	0-9421945513
• Patna	0-9334159340	• Pune	0-9923910676	• Uttarakhand	0-9716462459

Printed at   Gokul Offset Pvt. Ltd., Delhi (INDIA)

Foreword

The teachers of anatomy felt the need of a workbook for embryology for first MBBS students. This book is meant to sensitize the students regarding embryology models. The authors have taken care to include photographs of models of all the systems that students must know. The exercise of labelling models will make them understand and remember the development of each of the organs and at the same time prepare for the *viva voce* examination. This book in my opinion will be handy, useful and relevant to the requirements of the students to revise embryology. I hope it will make learning of human embryology simple and interesting.

My best wishes to the authors.

P Vatsalaswamy
Professor
Department of Anatomy
Director Academics
Dr DY Patil Medical College Hospital and
Research Centre, Pune

Foreword

It is a matter of pleasure and pride to pen foreword to this maiden endeavor of the authors who have taken all efforts to bring out this workbook. Understanding embryology has never been easy. It is a saga of events which happen over a time line. Students of first year MBBS usually find difficult to understand and remember the important embryological events in the process of development. Reinforcement of concepts understood is essential and that is where such workbooks step in. I am sure this workbook will reinforce the developmental facts and also clear the doubt in the minds of students so as to what will be expected of them in the practical examinations. I am sure this work will meet the desired goals.

My best wishes to the authors.

Purushottam Rao Manvikar
Professor and Head
Department of Anatomy
Dr DY Patil Medical College Hospital and
Research Centre, Pune

Preface

Embryology is one of the important parts of anatomy subject which first year MBBS students find difficult to cope up with, as they struggle to correlate various developmental processes along with new embryological terminology. Keeping this view in mind, this embryology workbook is made in systemwise manner which consists of not only actual photographs of embryo models but also some questions related to that particular model. Students will label the model and write answers to the questions in space provided during practical classes. This will enable students to understand and memorize the important developmental aspects of different systems of body, that will improve their performance in theory as well as *viva voce* examination in embryology. Also developing anatomy forms edifice of surgery, pediatrics branches so that undergraduates can also recapitulate developmental anomalies case scenarios. This book will be of great help to first MBBS students for remembering and revising the models effectively as well as related theory part.

This embryology workbook has been designed as per new competency based curriculum prescribed by Medical Council of India for Indian Medical Graduate.

Preeti Sonje
Neelesh Kanasker

Instructions for Students

- Students should label the photographs of the embryology model during embryology practical class.
- Labels of each photograph are indicated by numbers like 1, 2, 3, ... which the students are expected to know about that particular model.
- Students should label these numbers as well as write the answers of the questions asked in the space provided.

Contents

General Embryology

Cell Division—Mitosis

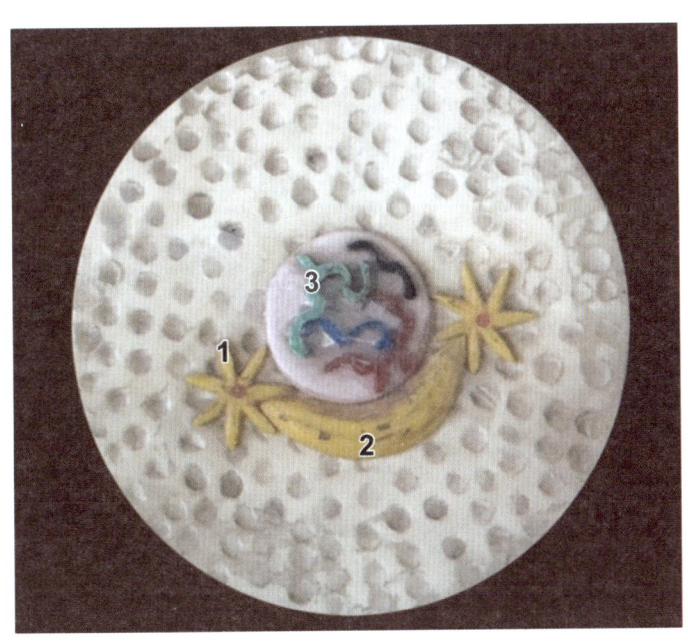

1. ....
   ....
2. ....
   ....
3. ....
   ....

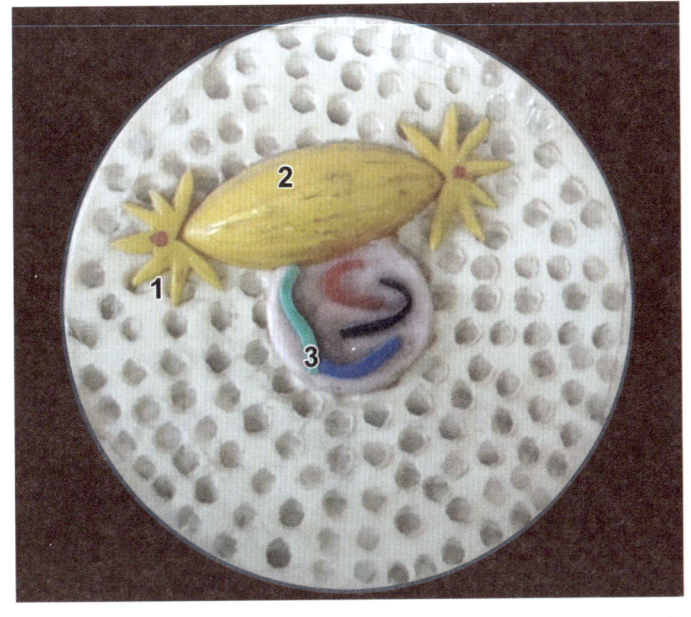

1. ....
   ....
2. ....
   ....
3. ....
   ....

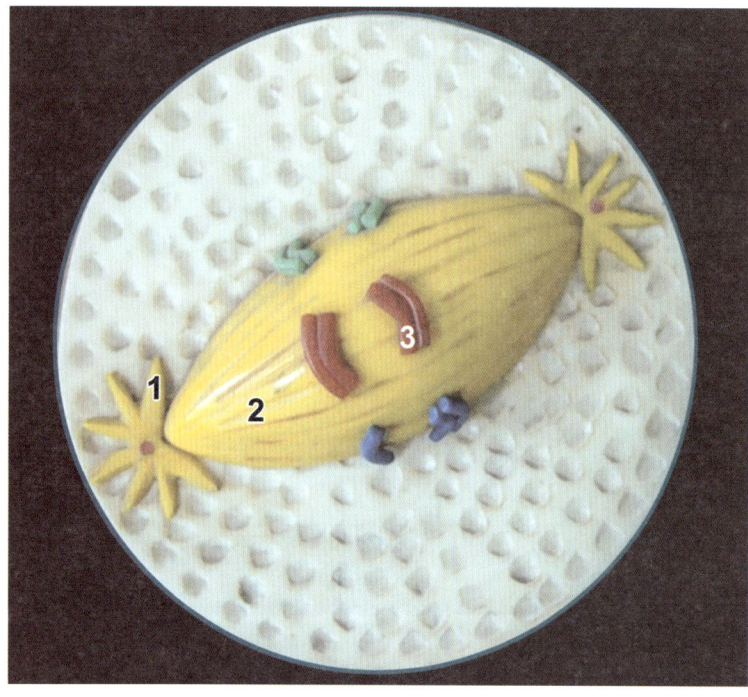

1. ....
   ....
2. ....
   ....
3. ....
   ....

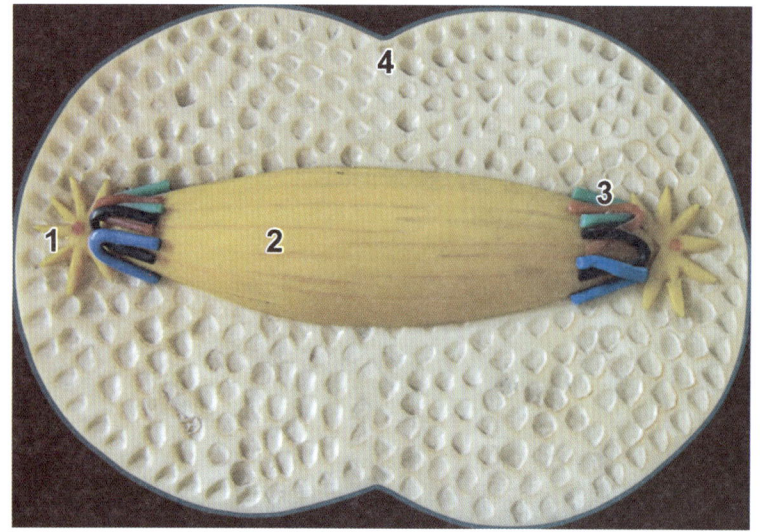

1. ....
   ....
2. ....
   ....
3. ....
   ....
4. ....
   ....

1. What are the types of cell division?

....

....

....

....

....

2. Write the differences between mitosis and meiosis.

3. What are the peculiarities of metaphase chromosomes?

....

....

....

....

....

4. What are the peculiarities of anaphase?

....

....

....

....

....

5. What is non-disjunction? What are its effects?

....

....

....

....

....

....

....

....

....

....

....

....

....

....

Spermatogenesis

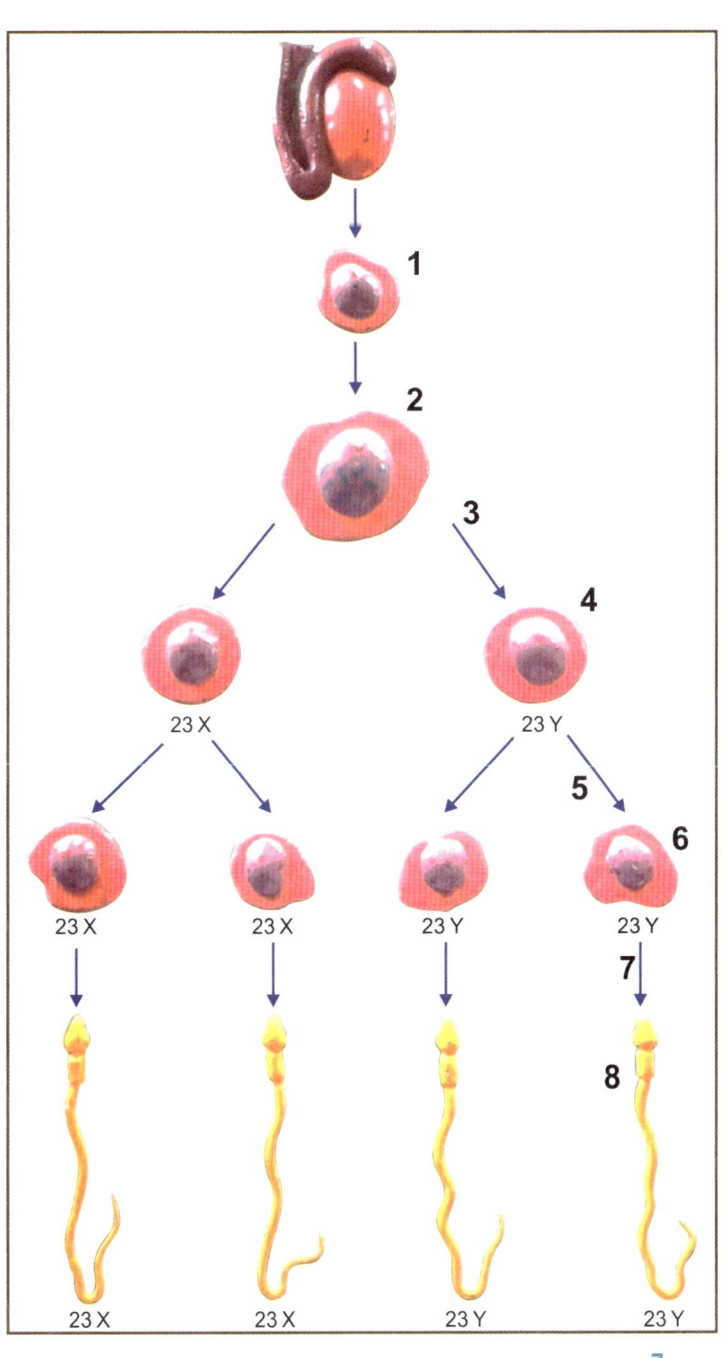

23 X   23 Y

23 X   23 X   23 Y   23 Y

23 X   23 X   23 Y   23 Y

1. ....
....
2. ....
....
3. ....
....
4. ....
....
5. ....
....
6. ....
....
7. ....
....
8. ....
....

1. What is spermatogenesis? When does it start?

....

....

....

....

2. When does the first meiotic division occur in spermatogenesis?

....

....

....

....

3. When does the second meiotic division occur in spermatogenesis?

....

....

....

....

4. Describe spermiogenesis.

....

....

....

....

5. What is oligozoospermia? Mention the causes of male infertility.

....

....

....

....

Maturation of Ovarian Follicle

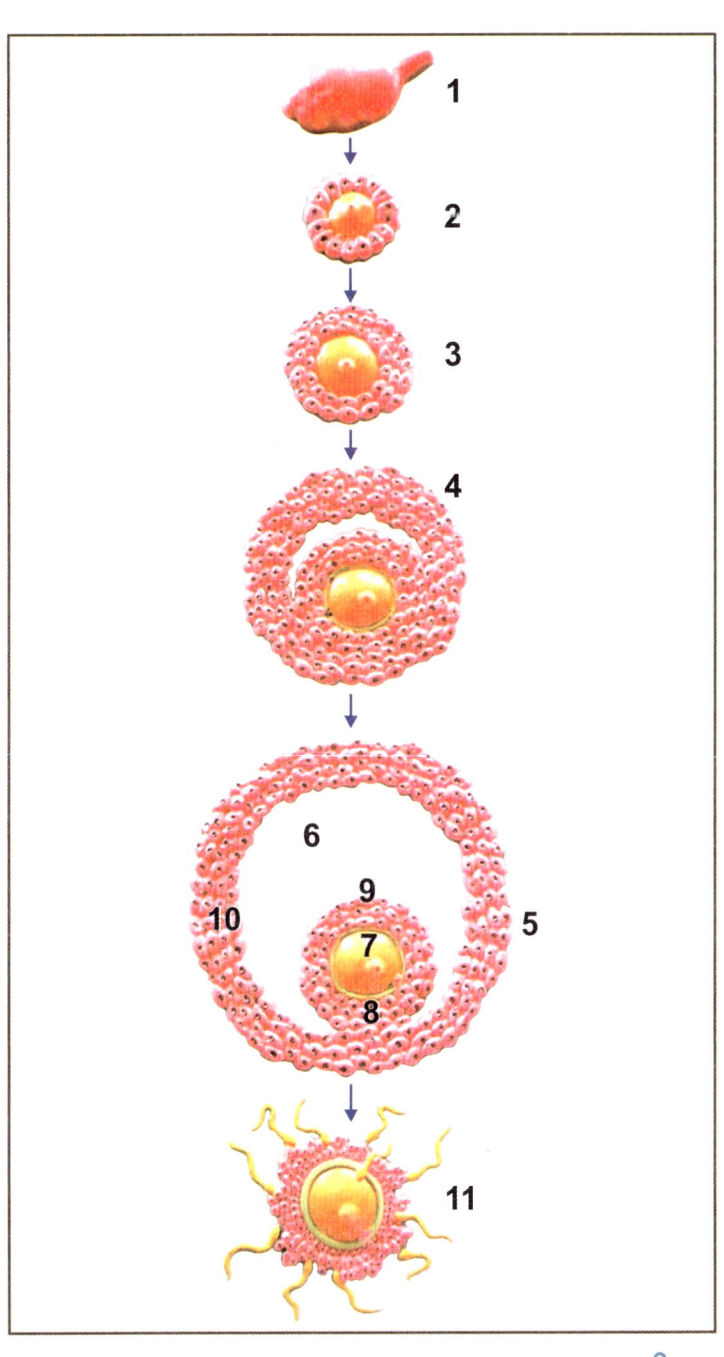

1. ....
....
2. ....
....
3. ....
....
4. ....
....
5. ....
....
6. ....
....
7. ....
....
8. ....
....
9. ....
....
10. ....
....
11. ....
....

1. When does the oogenesis start, at which phase it is arrested?

....

....

....

....

....

2. When does the first and second meiotic divisions take place in oogenesis?

....

....

....

....

....

3. What is polar body? What is its importance?

....

....

....

....

....

4. What is liquor folliculi?

....

....

....

....

....

Ovary

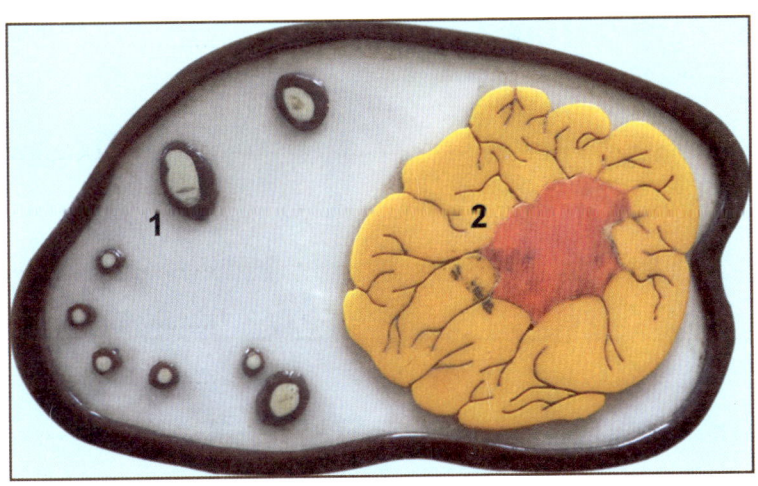

1. ....

2. ....

1. When does the oogenesis start, at which phase it is arrested?

....

....

....

....

2. How many number of ovarian follicles are present at the time of birth?

....

....

....

....

1. Describe the structure of:

a. Primordial follicle

....

....

....

b. Primary follicle

....

....

....

c. Secondary follicle

....

....

....

d. Graafian follicle

....

....

....

2. What is atretic follicle?

....

....

....

....

....

....

Corpus Luteum

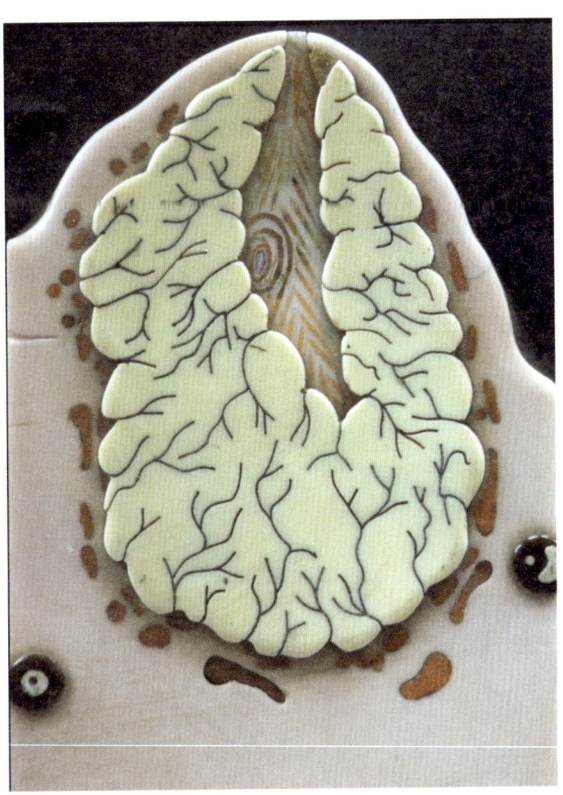

1. What is corpus luteum? How is it formed? Describe the structure of corpus luteum.

....

....

....

2. Mention the types of corpus luteum with their functions.

....

....

....

Ovulation and Implantation

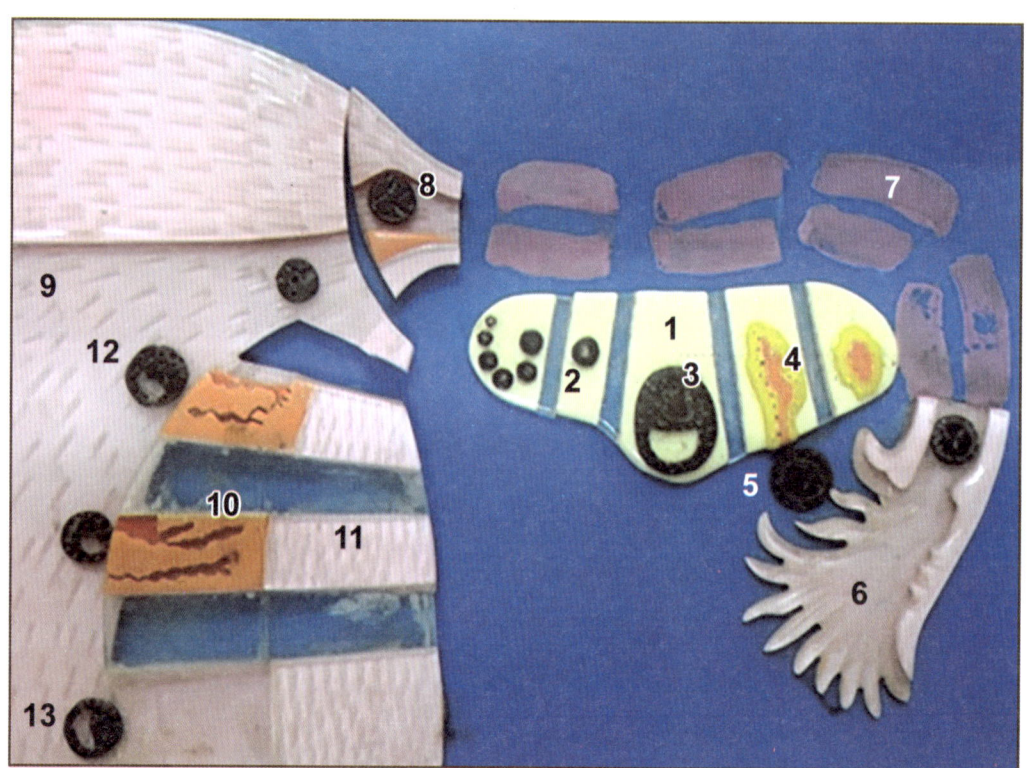

1. ....

2. ....

3. ....

4. ....

5. ....

6. ....

7. ....

8. ....

9. ....

10. ....

11. ....

12. ....

13. ....

1. What is an anovulatory cycle? Mention the causes of female infertility.

....

....

....

....

....

....

2. What is ovulation?

....

....

....

3. What is implantation?

....

....

....

4. Which is the commonest site of implantation?

....

....

....

5. Which hormones are required for implantation?

....

....

....

6. On which day implantation occurs?

....

....

....

7. What is ectopic pregnancy? Mention the sites of ectopic pregnancy.

....

....

....

Fertilization

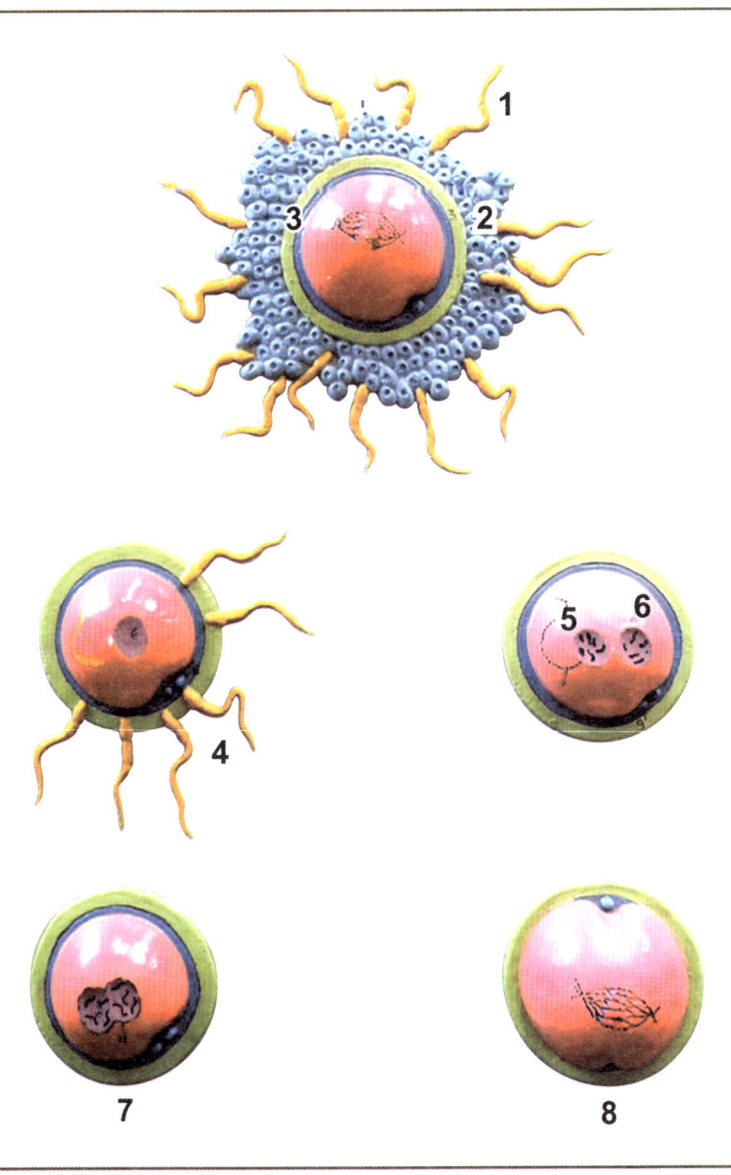

1. ....
....
2. ....
....
3. ....
....
4. ....
....
5. ....
....
6. ....
....
7. ....
....
8. ....
....

1. What is fertilization?

....

....

....

....

....

2. Mention the site of fertilization.

....

....

....

....

....

3. Describe the phases of fertilization.

....

....

....

....

....

....

....

....

....

....

....

....

....

4. What are the effects of fertilization?

....

....

....

....

....

....

....

....

....

....

....

....

....

....

....

Primary Chorionic Villi

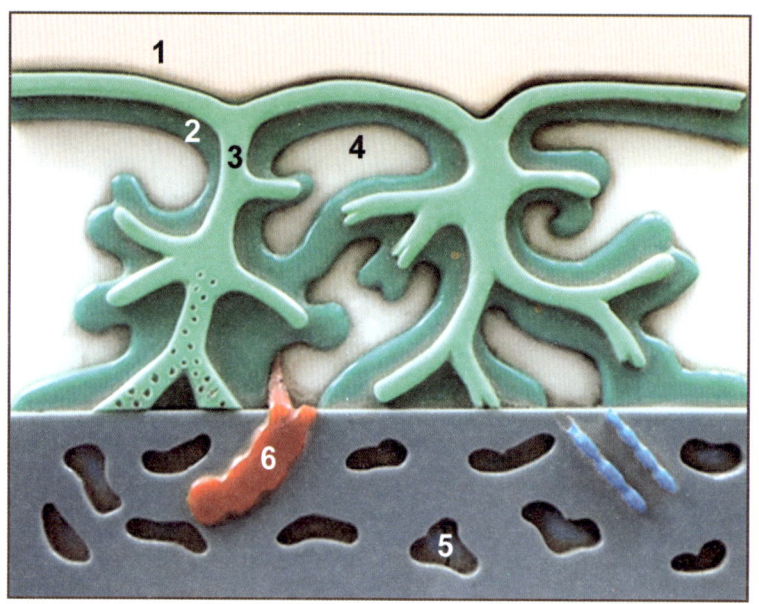

1. ....

2. ....

3. ....

4. ....

5. ....

6. ....

Secondary Chorionic Villi

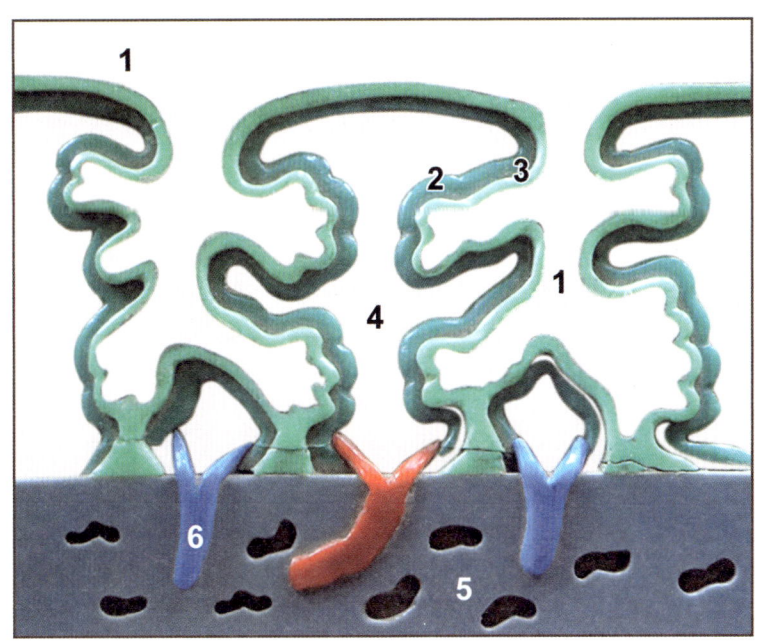

1. ....

2. ....

3. ....

4. ....

5. ....

6. ....

Tertiary Chorionic Villi

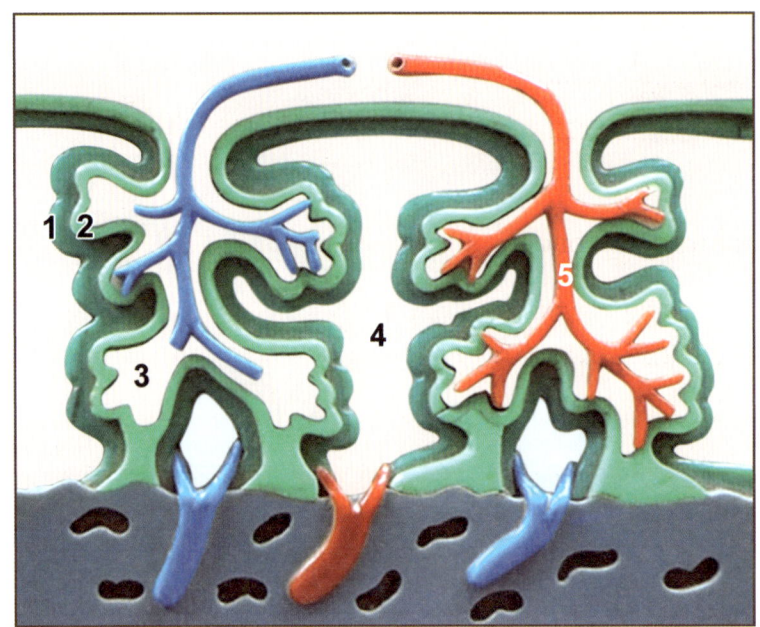

1. ....

2. ....

3. ....

4. ....

5. ....

1. Describe the structure of primary chorionic villus.

....
....
....
....
....
....
....

2. Describe the structure of secondary chorionic villus.

....
....
....
....
....
....
....

3. Describe the structure of tertiary chorionic villus.

....
....
....
....
....
....
....

Section of Placenta

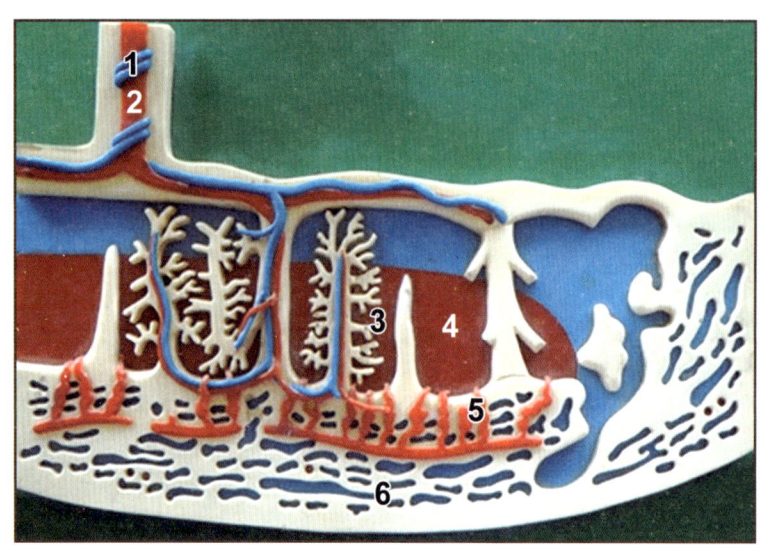

1. ....

2. ....

3. ....

4. ....

5. ....

6. ....

1. What is chorion?

....

....

....

2. What is decidua?

....

....

....

3. What are the functions of placenta?

....

....

....

4. What is placenta previa?

....

....

....

5. What are the components of placental barrier?

....

....

....

6. Enumerate the features of human placenta.

....

....

....

Blastocyst

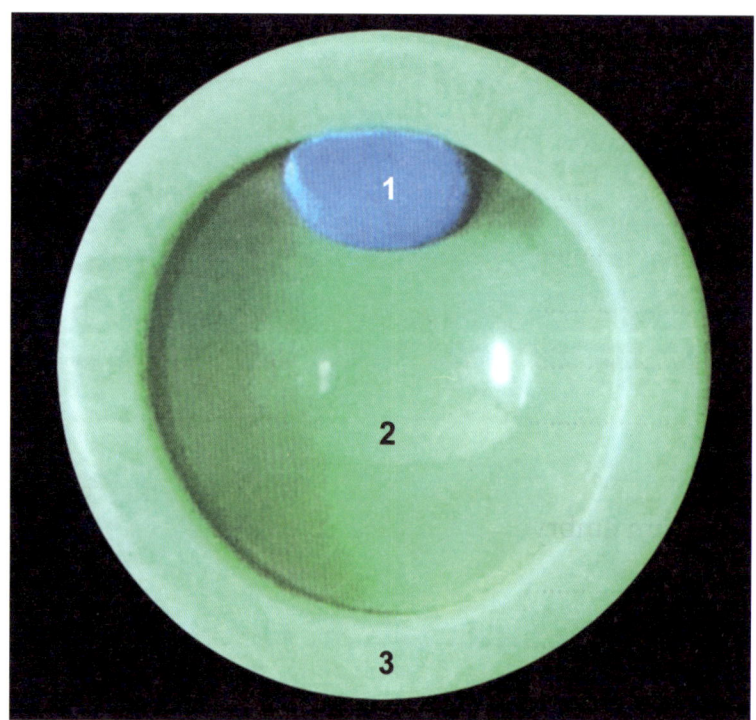

1. ....

2. ....

3. ....

1. What is embryoblast?

....
....
....
....
....

2. What is trophoblast?

....
....
....
....
....

3. What is developed from embryoblast?

....
....
....
....
....

4. What is developed from trophoblast?

....
....
....
....
....

Bilaminar Embryo

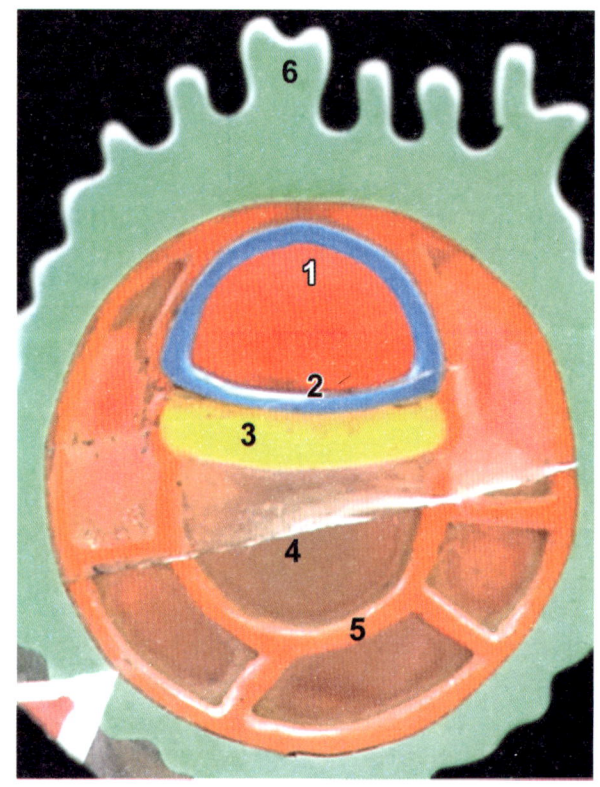

1. ....

2. ....

3. ....

4. ....

5. ....

6. ....

1. What does epiblast give rise to?

....
....
....
....

2. What does hypoblast give rise to?

....
....
....
....

3. What is Heuser's membrane?

....
....
....
....

4. What is function of yolk sac cavity?

....
....
....
....

5. What are amniogenic cells? What is their role?

....
....
....
....

Folding of Embryo I

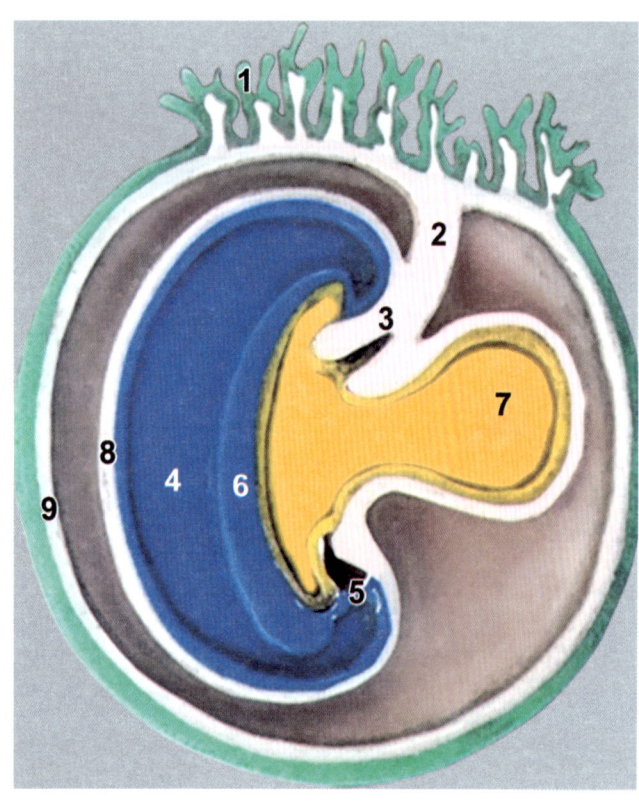

1. ....

2. ....

3. ....

4. ....

5. ....

6. ....

7. ....

8. ....

9. ....

1. What is allantoic diverticulum?

....

....

2. What is the fate of connecting stalk?

....

....

3. What is anterior intestinal portal?

....

....

4. What is posterior intestinal portal?

....

....

5. What is secondary yolk sac?

....

....

6. What is chorion frondosum?

....

....

7. What is chorion laeve?

....

....

15

Folding of Embryo II

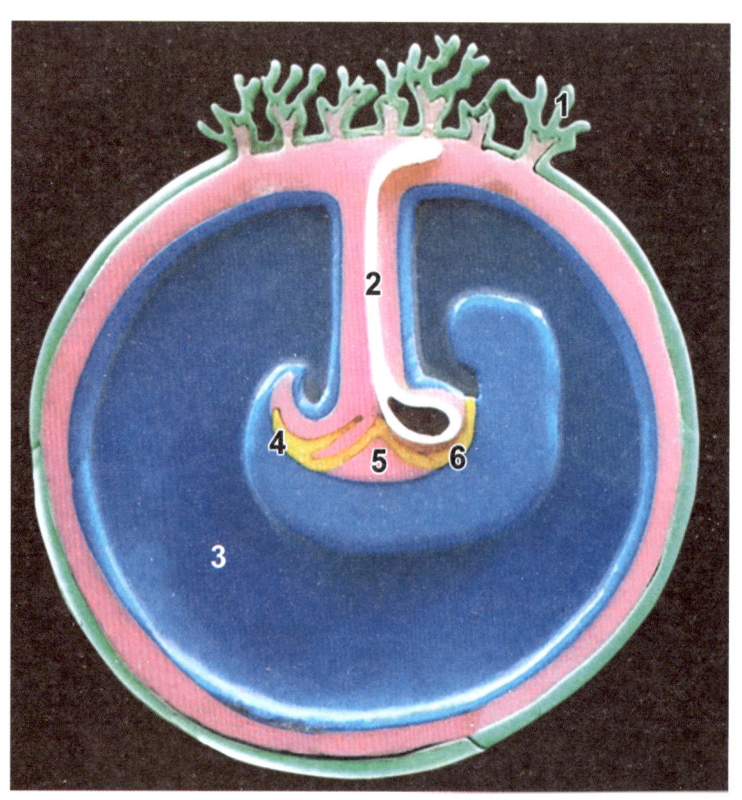

1. ....

2. ....

3. ....

4. ....

5. ....

6. ....

1. What is vitellointestinal duct?

....
....
....
....
....
....

2. What is Meckel's diverticulum?

....
....
....
....
....
....

3. What are the functions of amniotic cavity?

....
....
....
....
....
....

16

Trilaminar Embryo

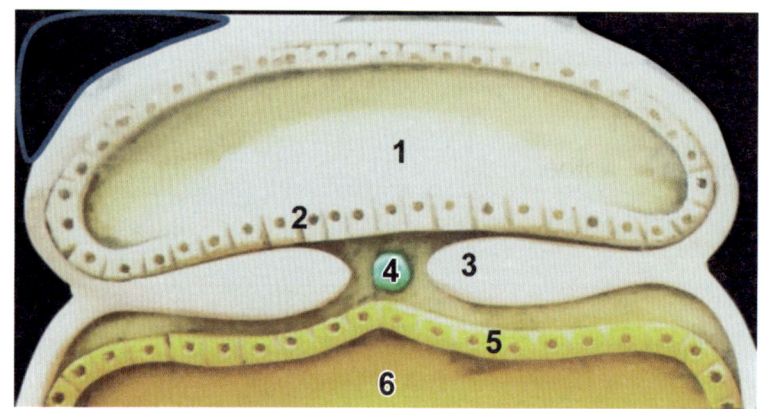

1. ....

2. ....

3. ....

4. ....

5. ....

6. ....

1. What is the function of notochord?

....

....

....

....

....

2. What are the remnants of notochord?

....

....

....

....

....

3. Name any five derivatives of ectoderm.

....

....

....

....

....

4. Name any five derivatives of endoderm.

....

....

....

....

....

Trilaminar Embryo with Neural Groove

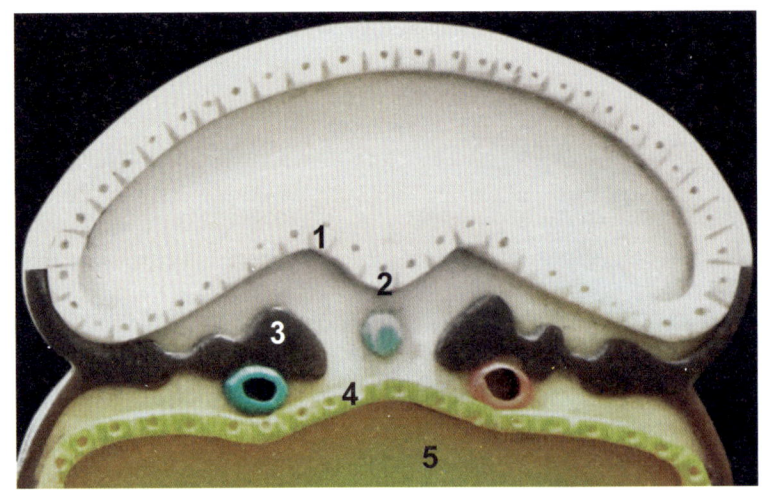

1. ....

2. ....

3. ....

4. ....

5. ....

Neurulation

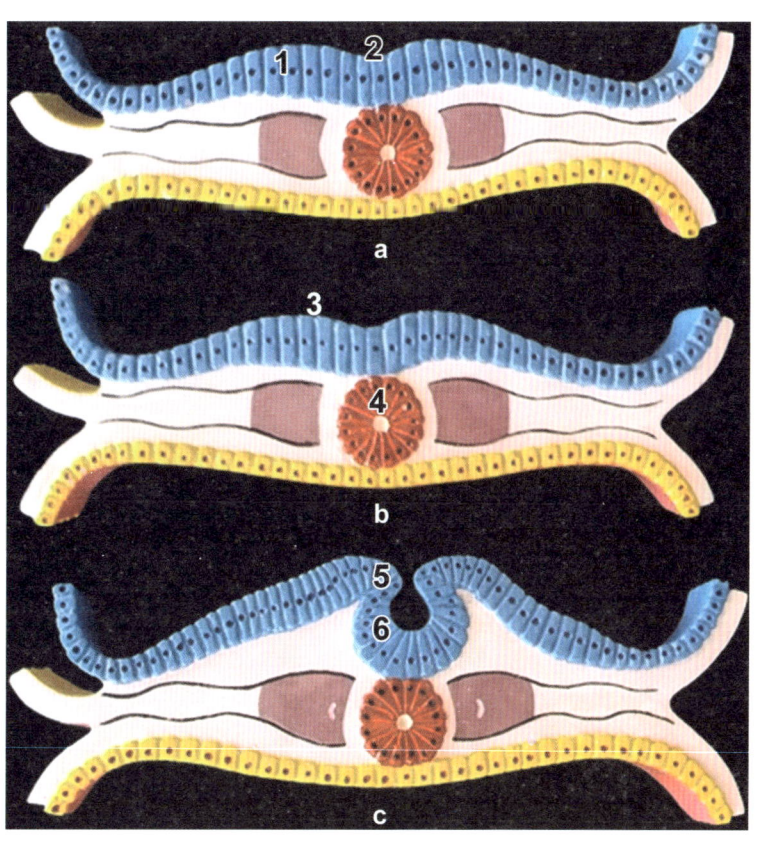

1. ....

2. ....

3. ....

4. ....

5. ....

6. ....

1. What is neurulation?

....

....

....

....

2. What is neural groove? Where does it appears?

....

....

....

....

3. What are neural folds?

....

....

....

....

4. What are neural crest cells?

....

....

....

....

5. Name any five derivatives of neural crest cells.

....

....

....

....

Trilaminar Embryo with Neural Tube

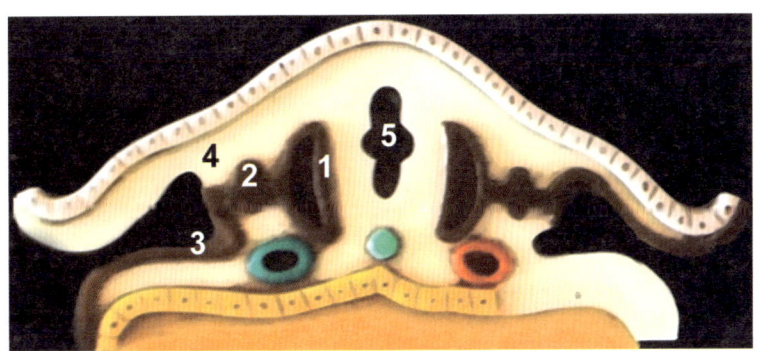

1. ....

2. ....

3. ....

4. ....

5. ....

1. Name the divisions of intraembryonic mesoderm.

....

....

....

....

2. What is derived from the neural tube?

....

....

....

....

3. What is derived from paraxial mesoderm?

....

....

....

....

4. What is derived from intermediate mesoderm?

....

....

....

....

5. What is derived from lateral plate mesoderm?

....

....

....

....

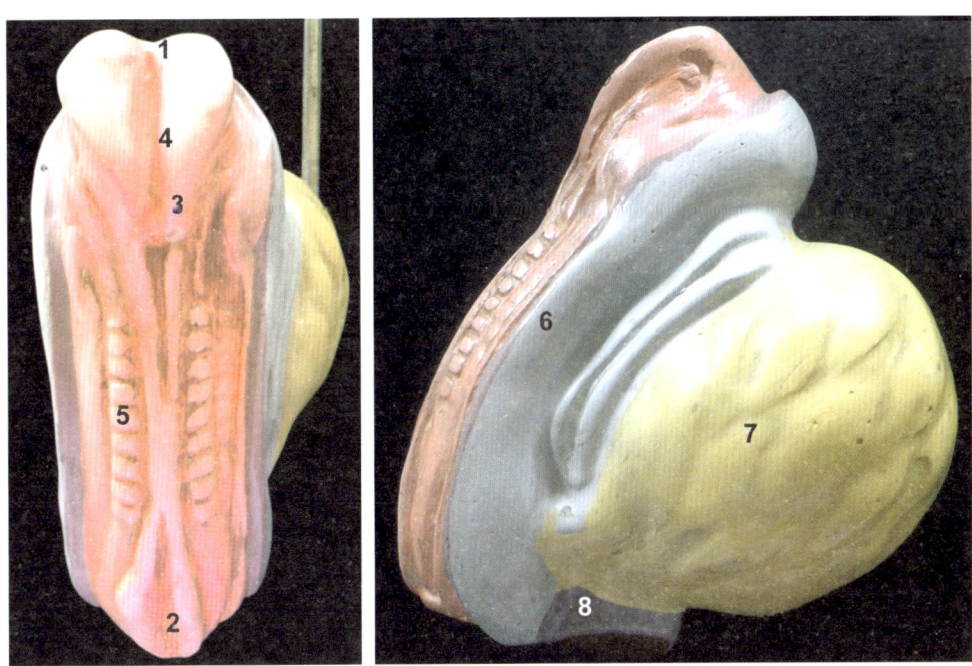

1. ....

2. ....

3. ....

4. ....

5. ....

6. ....

7. ....

8. ....

1. When does the anterior neuropore close?

....

....

....

....

2. When does the posterior neuropore close?

....

....

....

....

3. How many total somites are formed?

....

....

....

....

4. What does somites give rise to?

....

....

....

....

5. What does non-closure of anterior and posterior neuropore gives rise to?

....

....

....

....

II

Development of Head, Neck and Face

21

Pharyngeal Arches

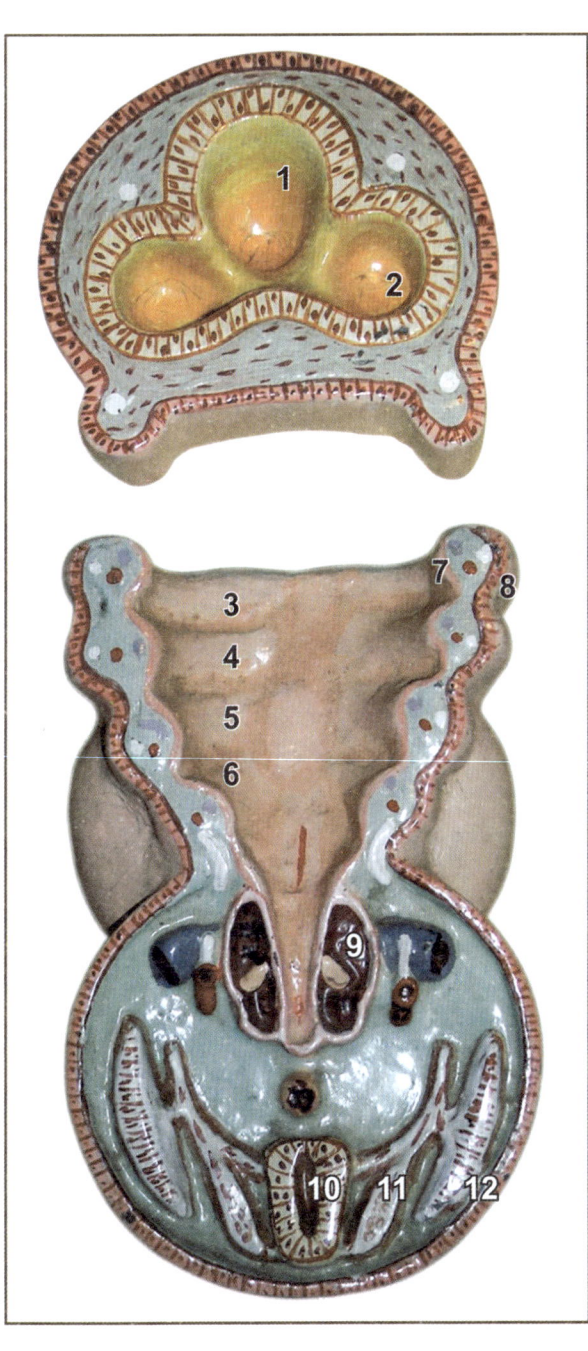

1. ....

2. ....

3. ....

4. ....

5. ....

6. ....

7. ....

8. ....

9. ....

10. ....

11. ....

12. ....

1. What are pharyngeal arches? How many pharyngeal arches are formed?

....

....

....

....

....

2. What are pharyngeal pouches?

....

....

....

....

....

3. What are pharyngeal clefts?

....

....

....

....

....

4. Mention all the derivatives of first pharyngeal arch.

....

....

....

....

....

5. Mention all the derivatives of second pharyngeal arch.

....

....

....

....

....

....

....

....

6. Mention all the derivatives of third pharyngeal arch.

....

....

....

....

....

....

....

....

7. Mention all the derivatives of fourth and sixth pharyngeal arches.

....

....

....

....

....

....

....

....

8. Name the nerves of all the pharyngeal arches.

....

....

....

....

....

....

....

....

....

....

9. Mention the derivatives of all the pharyngeal clefts.

....

....

....

....

....

....

....

....

....

....

22

Pharyngeal Pouches

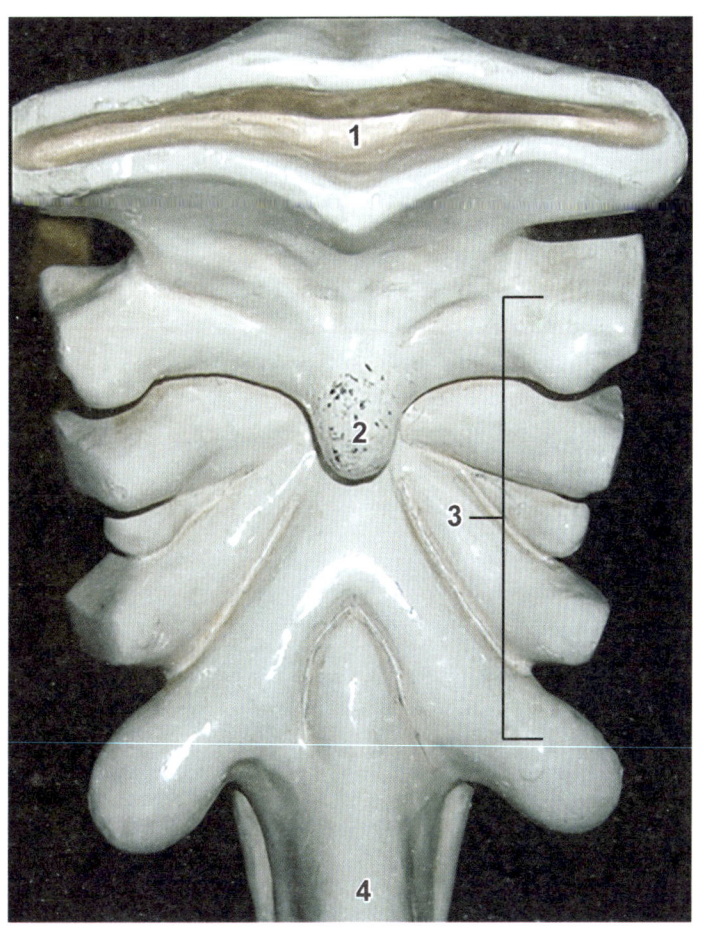

1. ....

2. ....

3. ....

4. ....

1. What are derivatives of 1st, 2nd, 3rd and 4th pharyngeal pouches?

....

....

....

....

....

....

....

....

2. What develops from thyroid diverticulum?

....

....

....

....

....

....

....

....

Development of Face

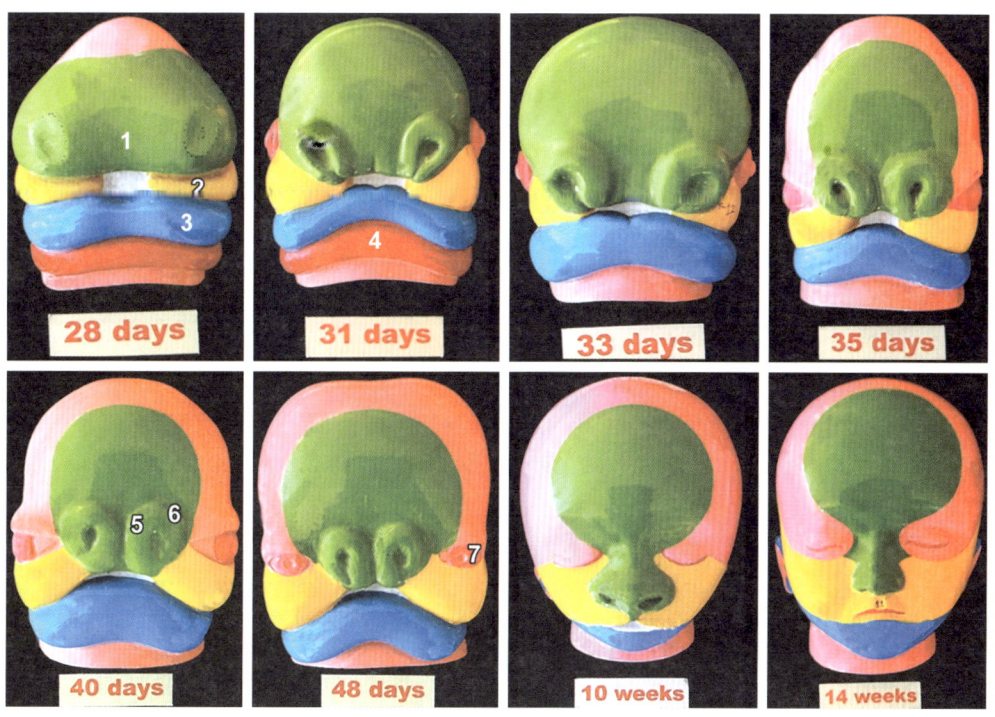

28 days • 31 days • 33 days • 35 days
40 days • 48 days • 10 weeks • 14 weeks

1. ....

2. ....

3. ....

4. ....

5. ....

6. ....

7. ....

1. Name the processes involved in the development of face.

....

....

....

....

....

....

....

....

2. Name the structures derived from the medial nasal process.

....

....

....

....

....

....

....

....

3. Name the different parts of face derived from different processes.

....

....

....

....

....

....

....

....

24 Development of Palate

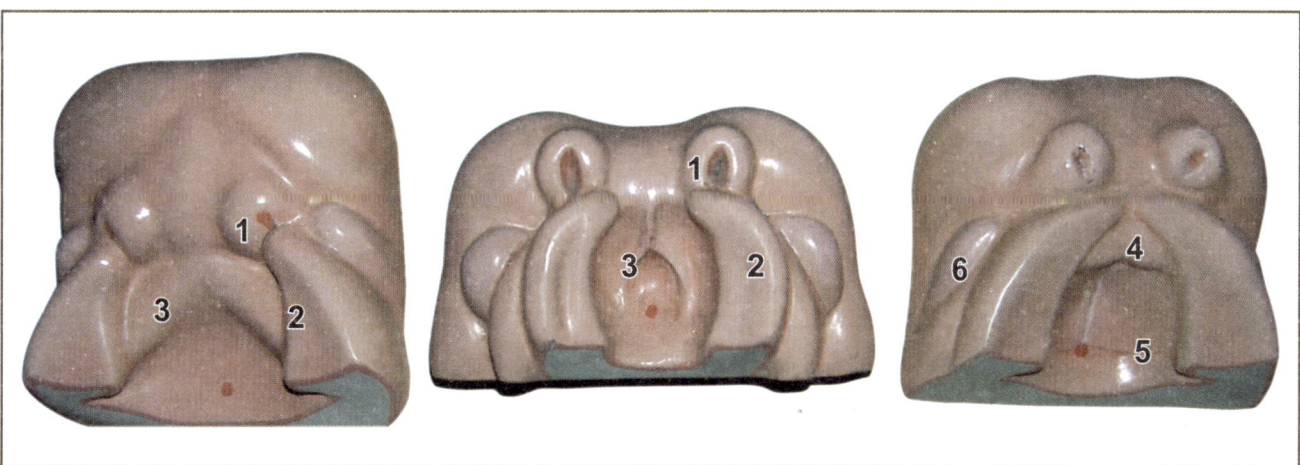

1. ....

2. ....

3. ....

4. ....

5. ....

6. ....

1. What is premaxilla?

....
....
....
....
....
....
....
....

2. What are palatine shelves?

....
....
....
....
....
....
....
....

3. What is cleft palate/hair lip? Mention its types.

....
....
....
....
....
....
....

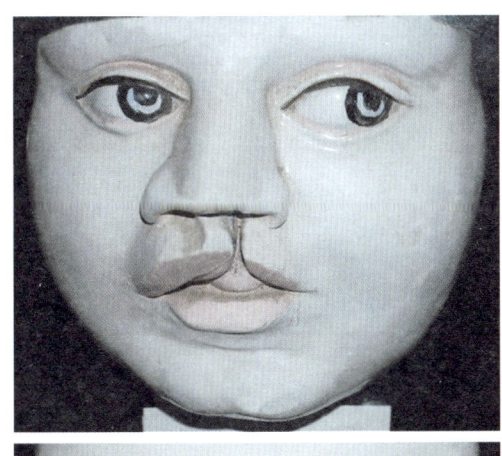

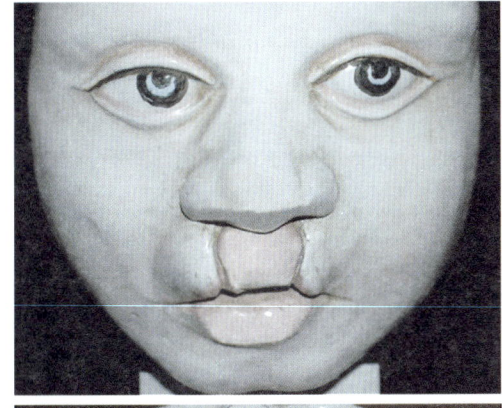

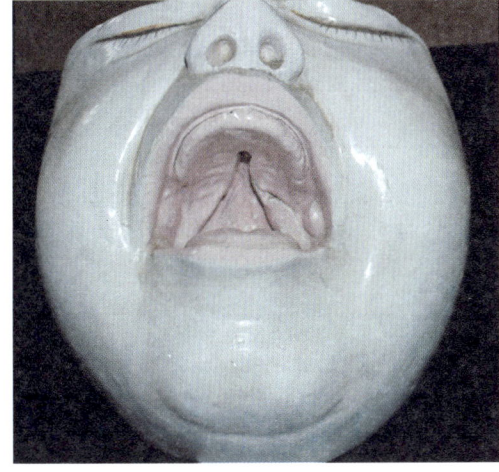

1. ....

2. ....

3. ....

1. What is embryological basis of nasolacrimal furrow?

....

....

....

....

....

....

....

....

2. What is embryological basis of cleft lip?

....

....

....

....

....

....

....

....

26

Development of Tongue

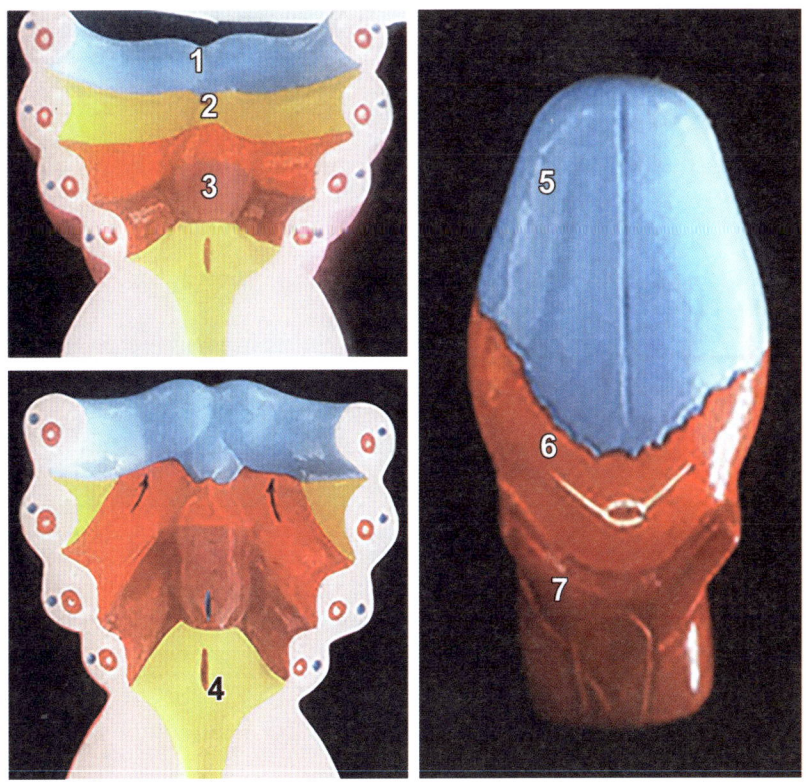

1. ....

2. ....

3. ....

4. ....

5. ....

6. ....

7. ....

1. Lingual swellings develop from which pharyngeal arch? What does it give rise to?

....

....

....

....

....

2. Hypobranchial eminence develop from which pharyngeal arch? What does it give rise to?

....

....

....

....

....

3. What is sulcus terminalis?

....

....

....

....

....

4. Name some developmental anomalies of tongue.

....

....

....

....

....

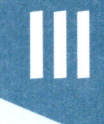

Development of Nervous System

27

Development of Spinal Cord

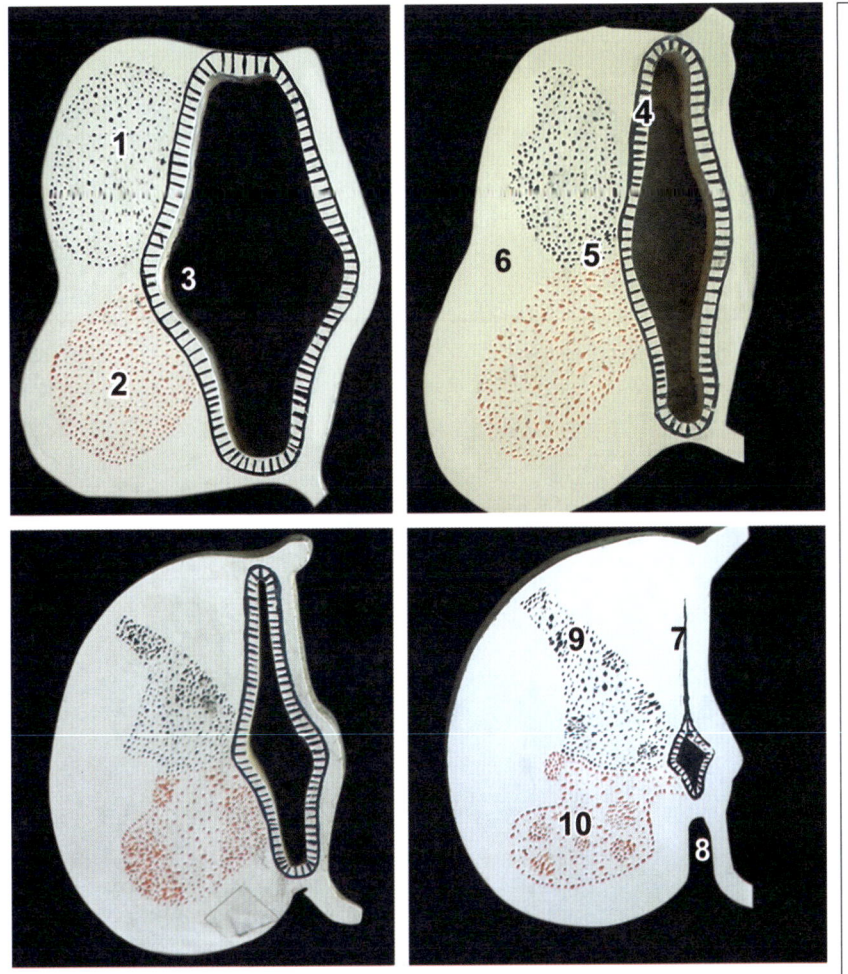

1. ....

2. ....

3. ....

4. ....

5. ....

6. ....

7. ....

8. ....

9. ....

10. ....

1. What are the three different layers of neural tube formed during development of spinal cord?

....

....

....

....

2. What is derived from alar lamina?

....

....

....

....

3. What is derived from basal lamina?

....

....

....

....

4. What is present in marginal layer?

....

....

....

....

5. What is present in mantle layer?

....

....

....

....

28

Development of Medulla, Pons and Cerebellum

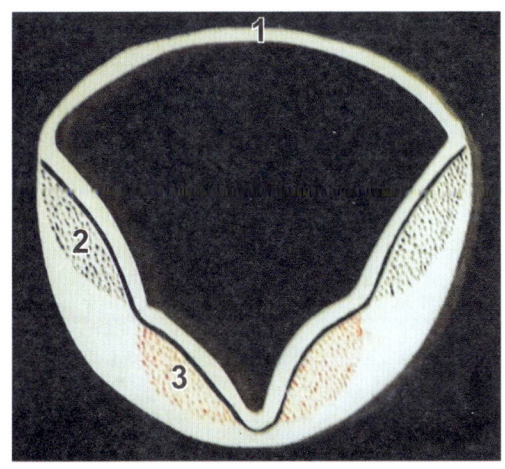

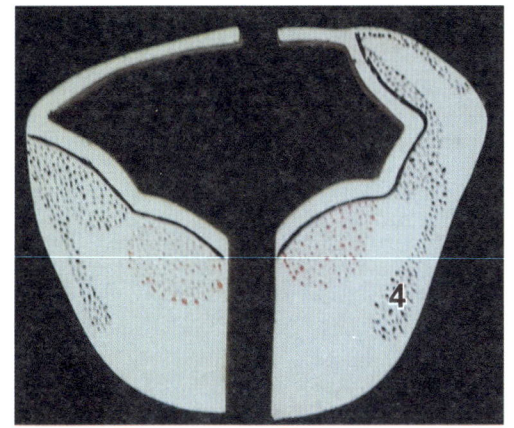

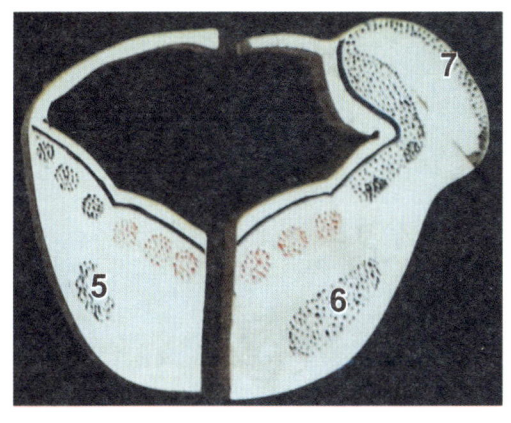

1. ....

2. ....

3. ....

4. ....

5. ....

6. ....

7. ....

1. What does bulbopontine extension give rise to?

....

....

....

....

....

....

....

....

2. What is formed from rhombic lip?

....

....

....

....

....

....

....

....

3. What are various functional components of cranial nerves?

....

....

....

....

....

....

....

....

IV

Development of Cardiovascular System

29

Development of Interatrial Septum

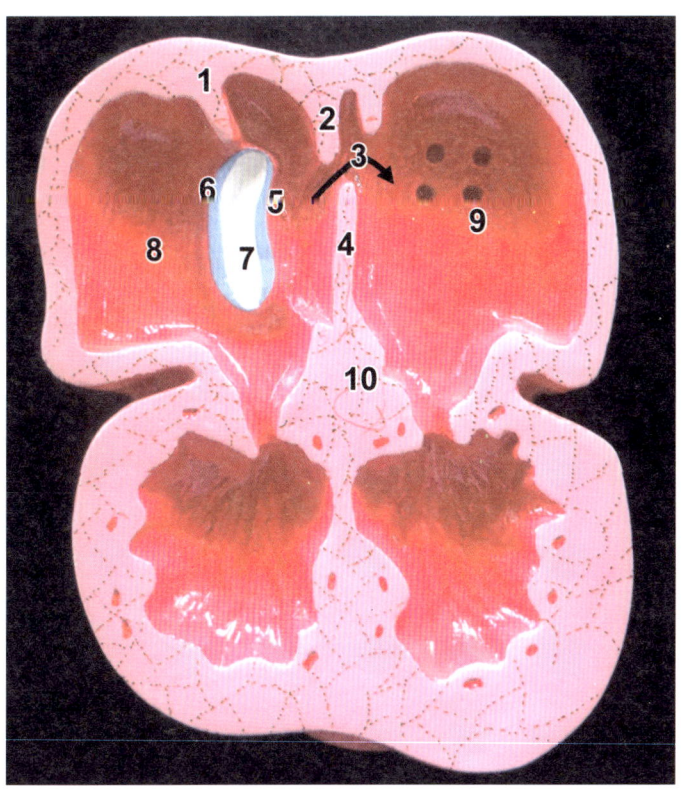

1. ....

2. ....

3. ....

4. ....

5. ....

6. ....

7. ....

8. ....

9. ....

10. ....

1. What are the developmental components of interatrial septum?

....

....

....

....

2. What is derived from right venous valve?

....

....

....

....

3. What is the remnant of septum primum?

....

....

....

....

4. What is the remnant of septum secondum?

....

....

....

....

5. What is foramen ovale and when does it close? What causes its closure?

....

....

....

....

6. What is atrial septal defect?

....

....

....

....

7. What is Fallot's tetralogy?

....

....

....

....

8. What is probe patency of foramen ovale?

....

....

....

....

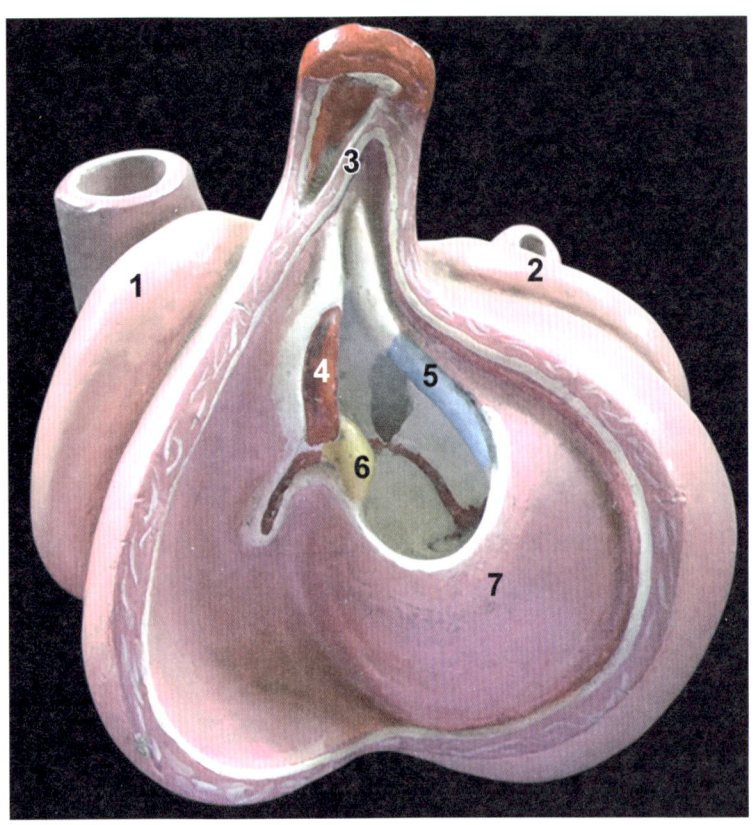

1. ....

2. ....

3. ....

4. ....

5. ....

6. ....

7. ....

1. What are the developmental components of interventricular septum?

....
....
....
....

2. What is the source of membranous part?

....
....
....
....

3. What is the source of muscular part?

....
....
....
....

4. What is ventricular septal defect? Mention its cause and types.

....
....
....
....
....
....
....

31

Aortic Arches

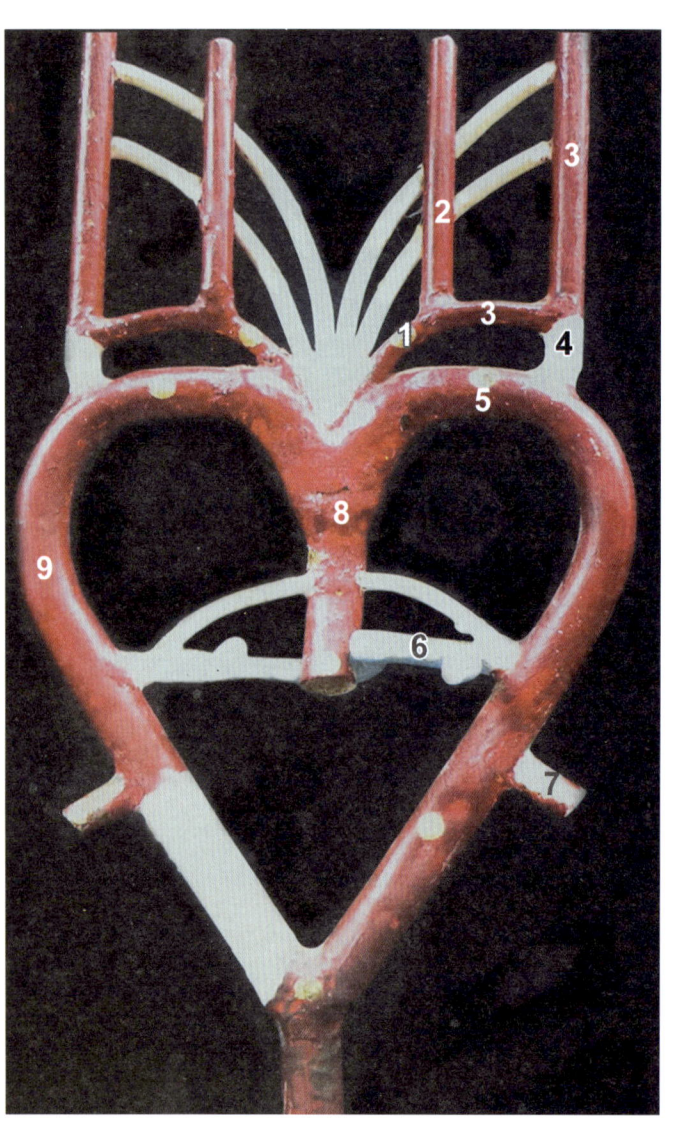

1. ....
....
2. ....
....
3. ....
....
4. ....
....
5. ....
....
6. ....
....
7. ....
....
8. ....
....
9. ....
....

1. What is derived from the third aortic arch?

....

....

....

2. What does the fourth aortic arch give rise to?

....

....

....

3. Mention the derivatives of sixth aortic arch.

....

....

....

4. What does seventh intersegmental artery give rise to?

....

....

....

5. What is the fate of ductus caroticus?

....

....

....

6. What is coarctation of aorta?

....

....

....

32

Development of Inferior Vena Cava

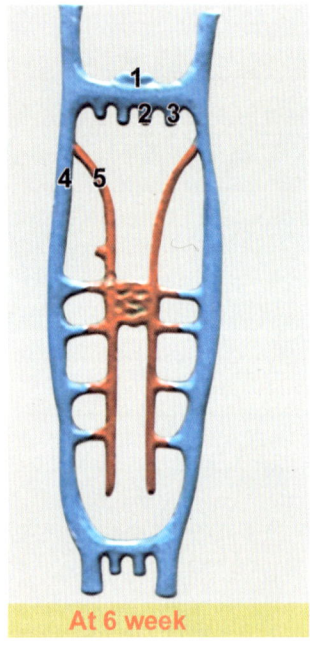

At 6 week

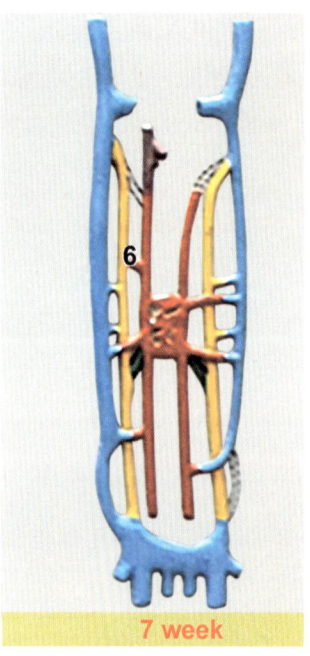

7 week

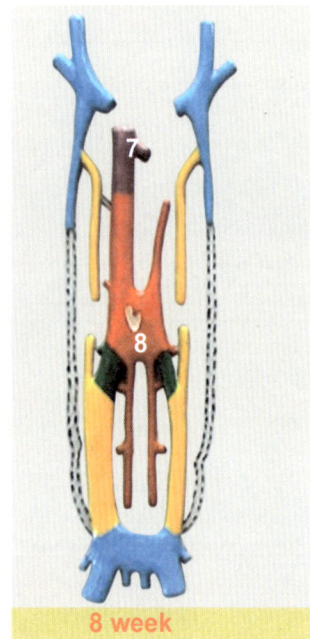

8 week

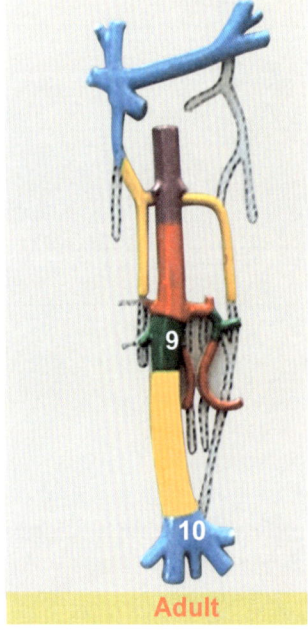

Adult

1. ....
....
2. ....
....
3. ....
....
4. ....
....
5. ....
....
6. ....
....
7. ....
....
8. ....
....
9. ....
....
10. ....
....

1. Mention the developmental components of inferior vena cava.

....

....

....

....

....

....

2. Name the veins that open into the sinus venosus?

....

....

....

....

....

....

33

Foetal Circulation

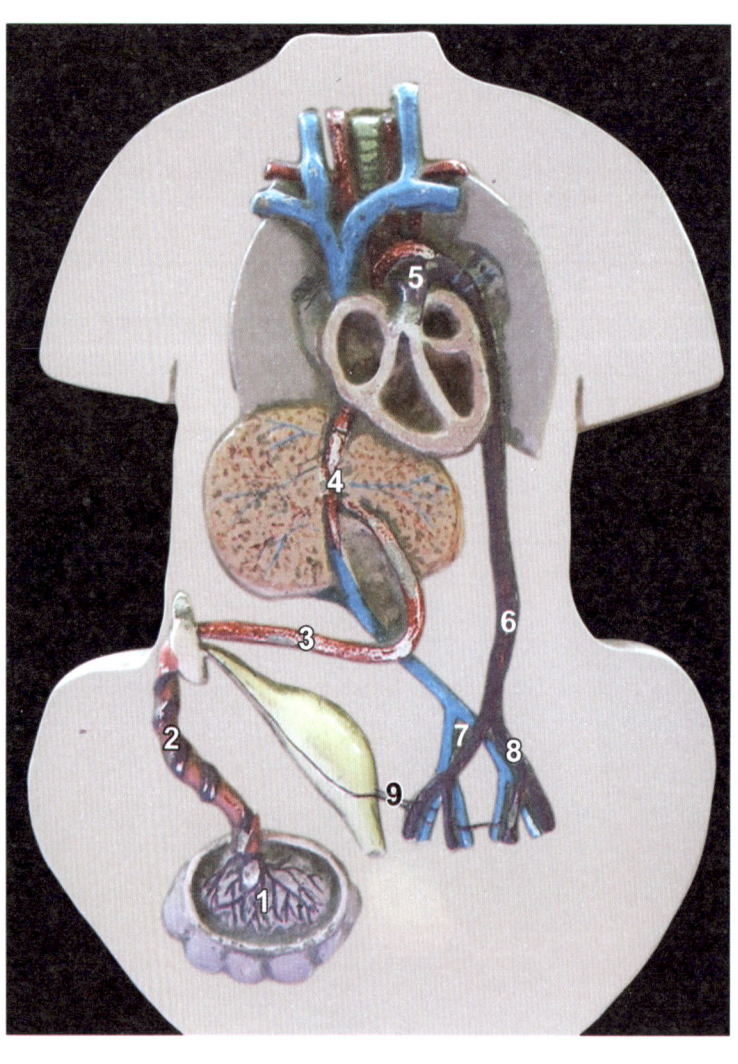

1. ....

2. ....

3. ....

4. ....

5. ....

6. ....

7. ....

8. ....

9. ....

1. What is ductus arteriosus? What is patent ductus arteriosus?

....

....

....

....

....

2. What is ductus venosus?

....

....

....

....

....

3. What is the fate of umbilical arteries?

....

....

....

....

....

4. What are the changes seen in foetal circulation after birth?

....

....

....

....

....

V

Development of Gastrointestinal Tract

Section of Abdominal Cavity of Embryo

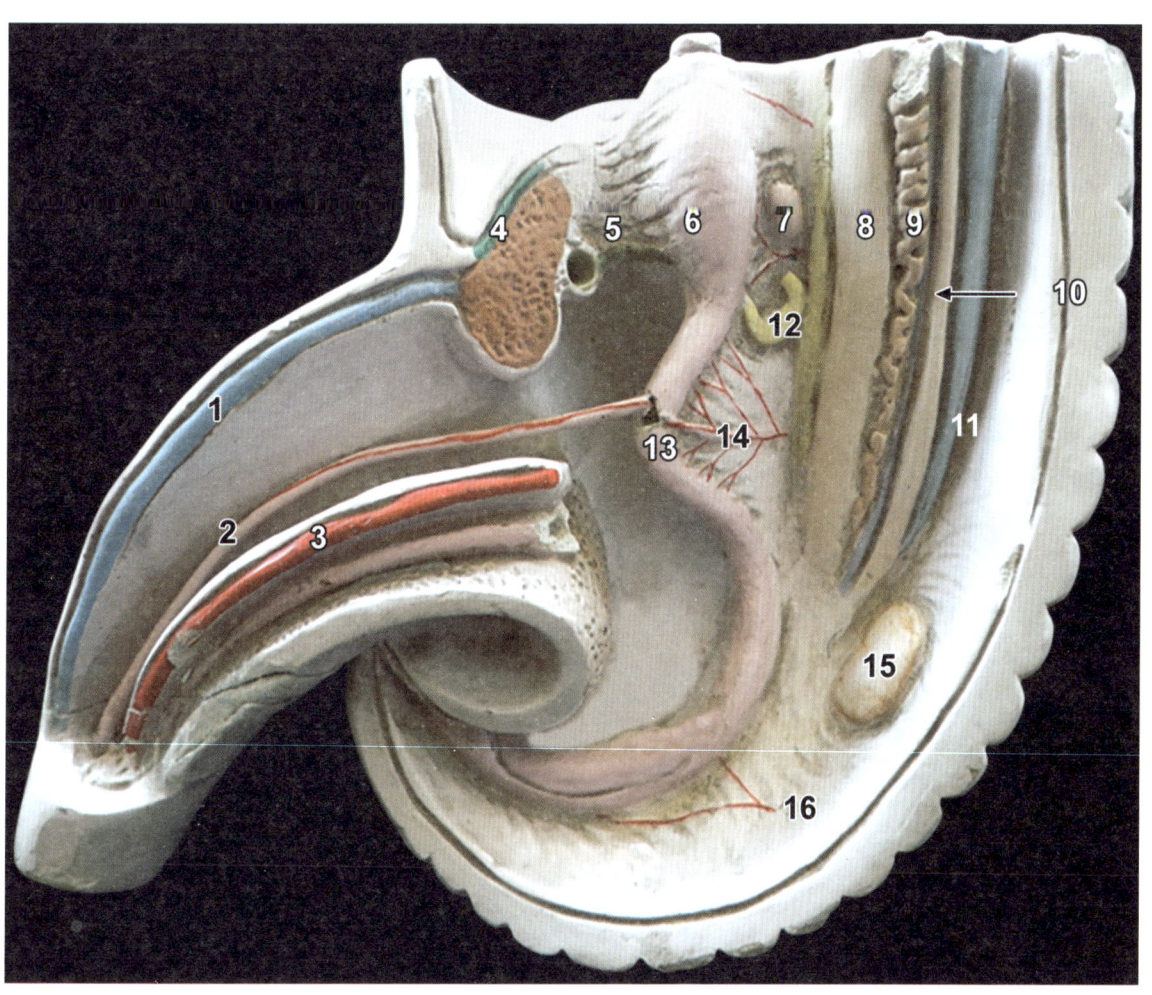

1. ....

2. ....

3. ....

4. ....

5. ....

6. ....

7. ....

8. ....

9. ....

10. ....

11. ....

12. ....

13. ....

14. ....

15. ....

16. ....

1. What are the derivatives of foregut?

....

....

....

....

....

2. Mention the derivatives of midgut.

....

....

....

....

....

3. What are the derivatives of hindgut?

....

....

....

....

....

4. Name the arteries of foregut, midgut and hindgut.

....

....

....

....

....

5. What develops in ventral mesogastrium and in dorsal mesogastrium?

....

....

....

....

....

....

6. What is vitellointestinal duct?

....

....

....

....

....

....

7. What is allantois?

....

....

....

....

....

....

35

Development of Pancreas

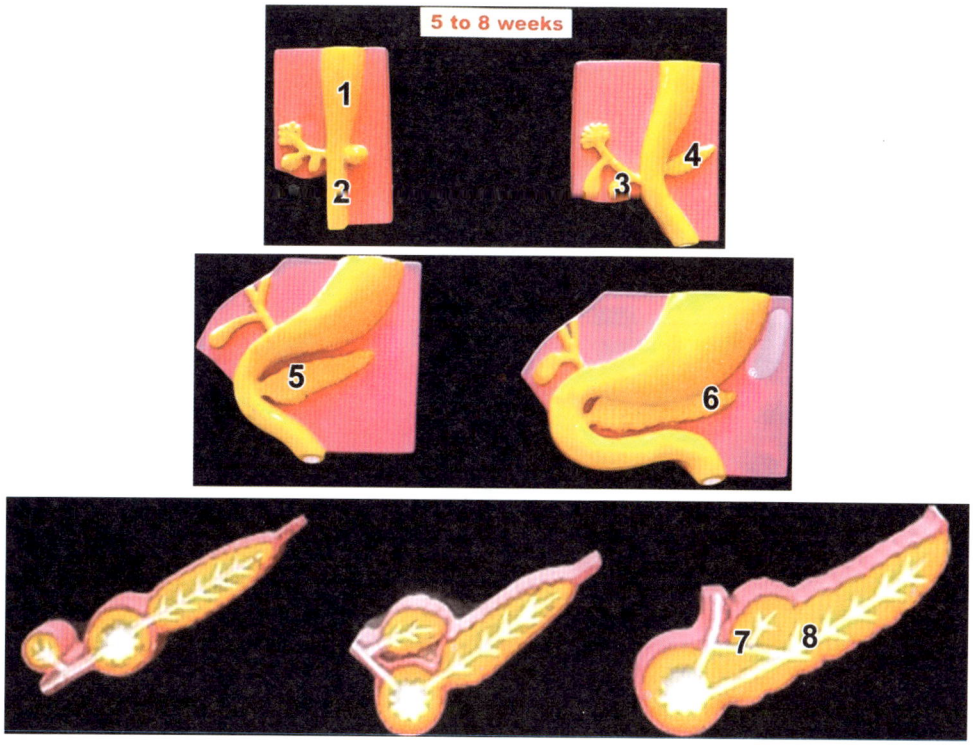

5 to 8 weeks

1. ....
2. ....
3. ....
4. ....
5. ....
6. ....
7. ....
8. ....

1. Mention the site of development of pancreas.

....

....

....

....

2. Which pancreatic bud undergoes rotation? Why?

....

....

....

....

3. Mention the parts of pancreas derived from dorsal and ventral pancreatic buds.

....

....

....

....

4. Which duct gives rise to the main pancreatic duct and accessory pancreatic duct?

....

....

....

....

5. What is annular pancreas?

....

....

....

....

36

Rotation of Midgut Loop

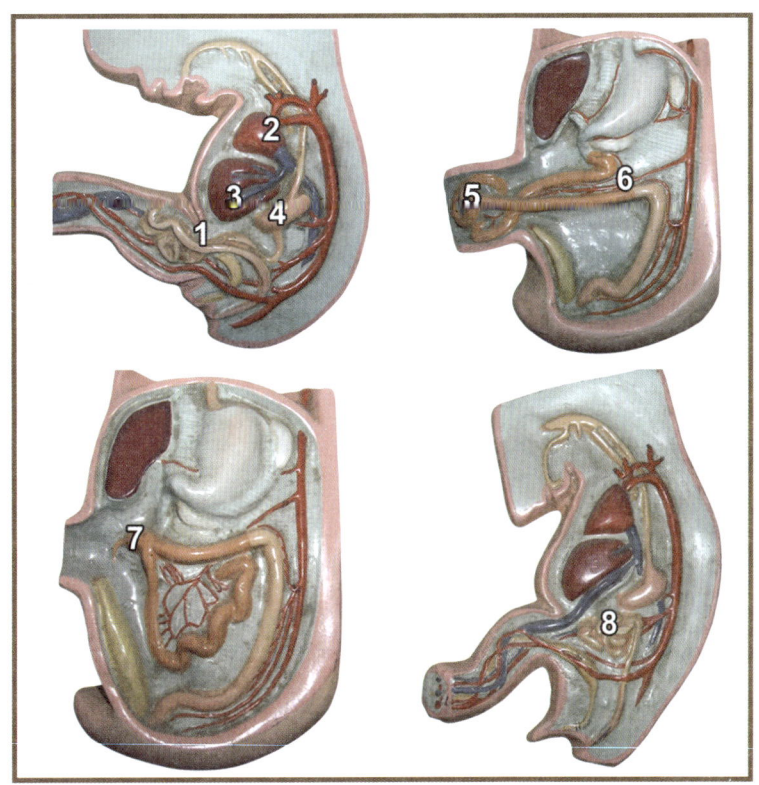

1. ....

2. ....

3. ....

4. ....

5. ....

6. ....

7. ....

8. ....

1. Which part of intestine is derived from prearterial segment?

....

....

....

....

....

2. Which part of intestine is derived from postarterial segment?

....

....

....

....

....

3. What is physiological umbilical hernia?

....

....

....

....

....

4. What are the causes of physiological umbilical hernia?

....

....

....

....

....

5. How much degree of total rotation of midgut loop takes place?

....

....

....

....

....

6. What is reduction of hernia?

....

....

....

....

....

7. What is Meckel's diverticulum?

....

....

....

....

....

8. What is omphalocele? What is gastroschisis?

....

....

....

....

....

Development of Caecum and Appendix

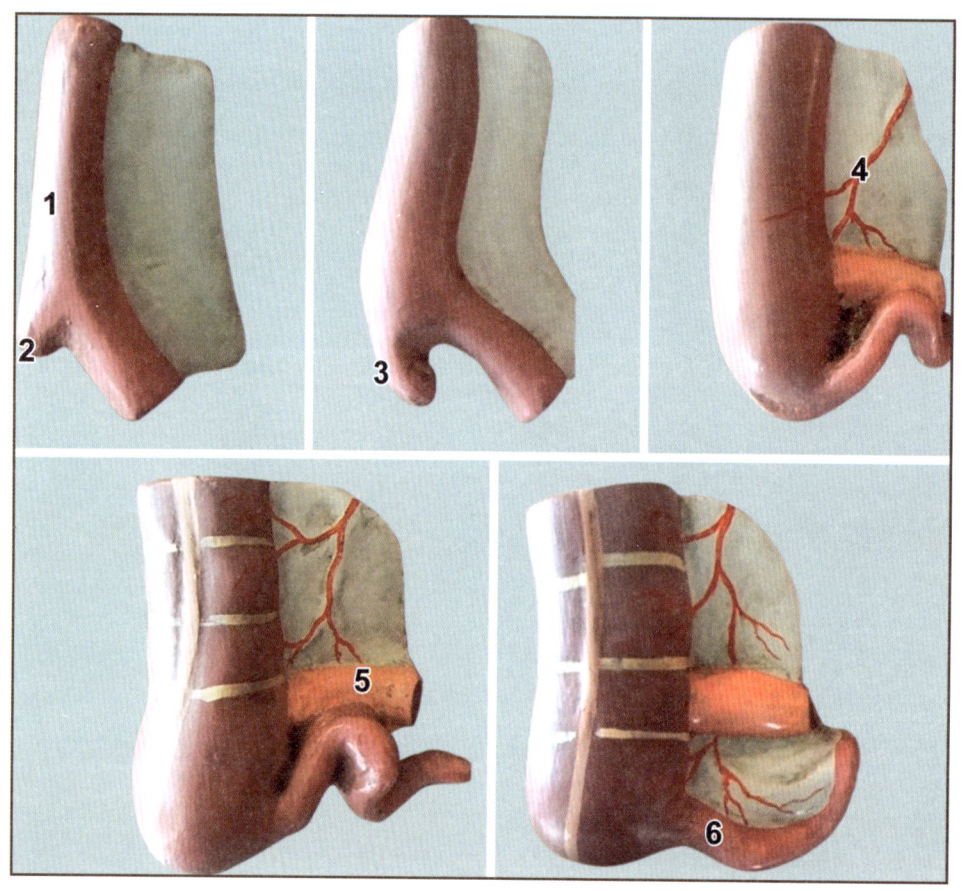

1. ....
2. ....
3. ....
4. ....
5. ....
6. ....

VI

Development of Urinary System

Development of Ureter

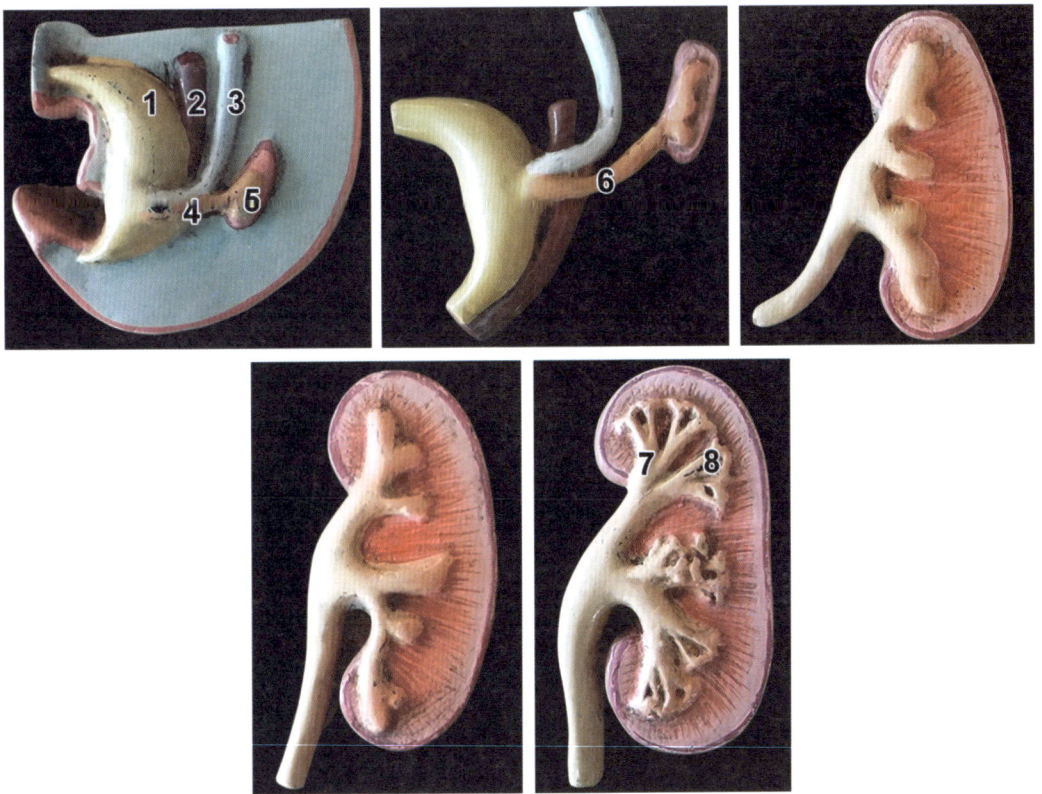

1. ....

2. ....

3. ....

4. ....

5. ....

6. ....

7. ....

8. ....

1. Which part of intraembryonic mesoderm gives rise to the urinary system?

....

....

....

....

2. How does ureter develop?

....

....

....

....

3. What are the two divisions of urogenital sinus? What are the structures derived from them?

....

....

....

....

4. What is metanephric blastema?

....

....

....

....

5. Name some developmental anomalies of kidney and ureter.

....

....

....

....

39

Development of Excretory Part of Kidney

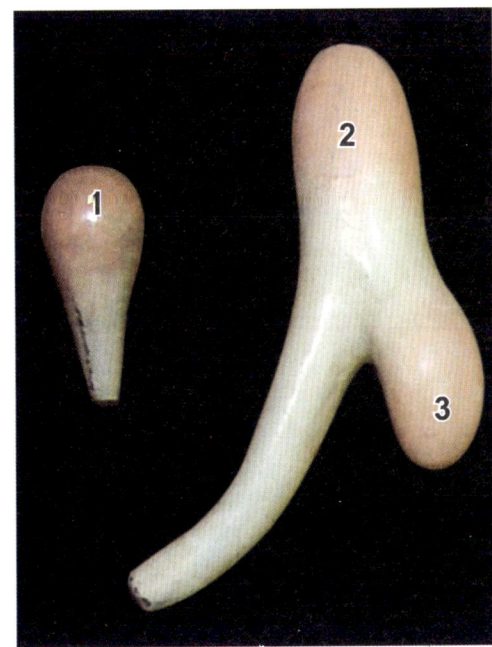 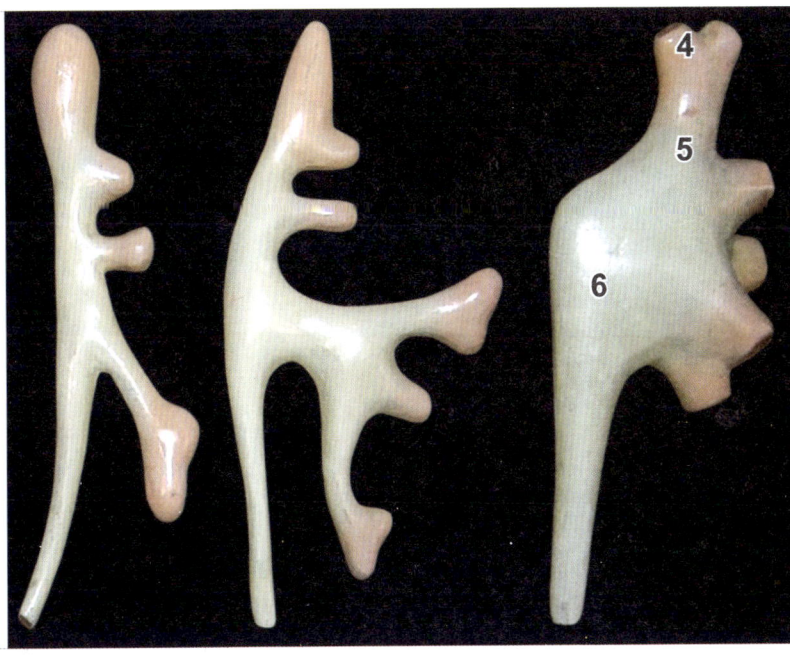

1. ....

2. ....

3. ....

4. ....

5. ....

6. ....

40 Anomalies of Urachus

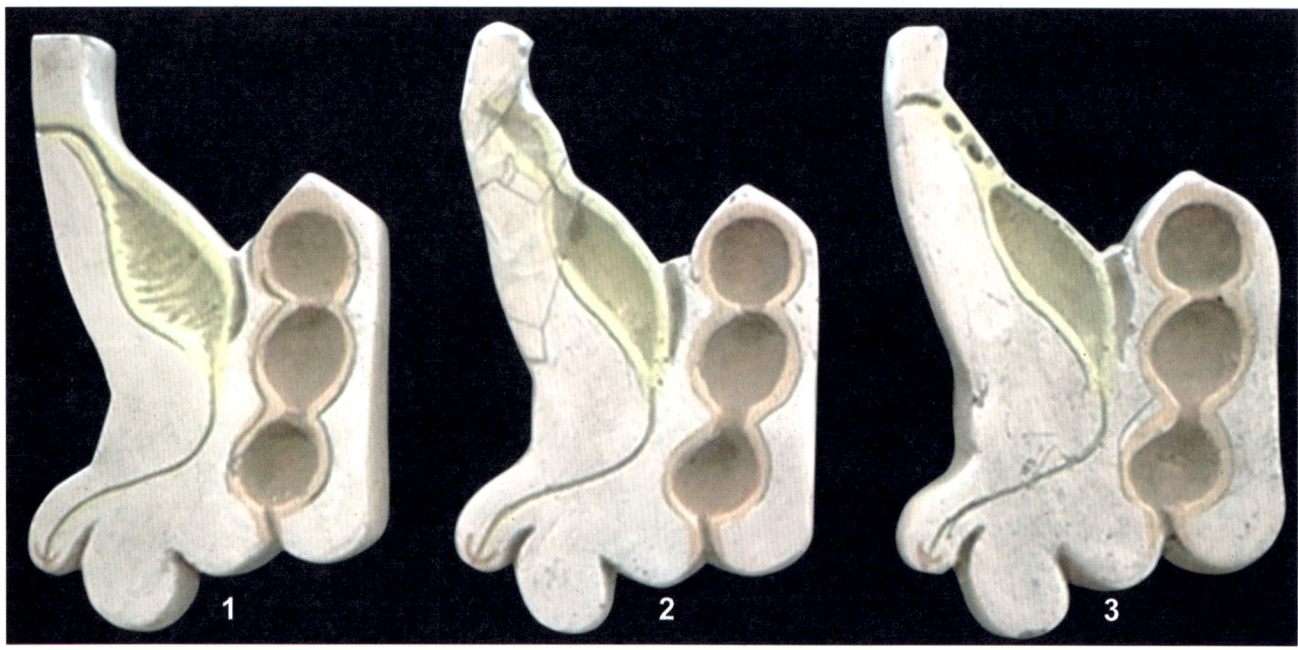

1

2

3

---

1. ....

2. ....

3. ....

---

1. What is urachus?

....

....

2. What is ectopia vesicae?

....

....

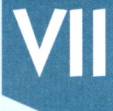

Development of Reproductive System

Development of Gonads

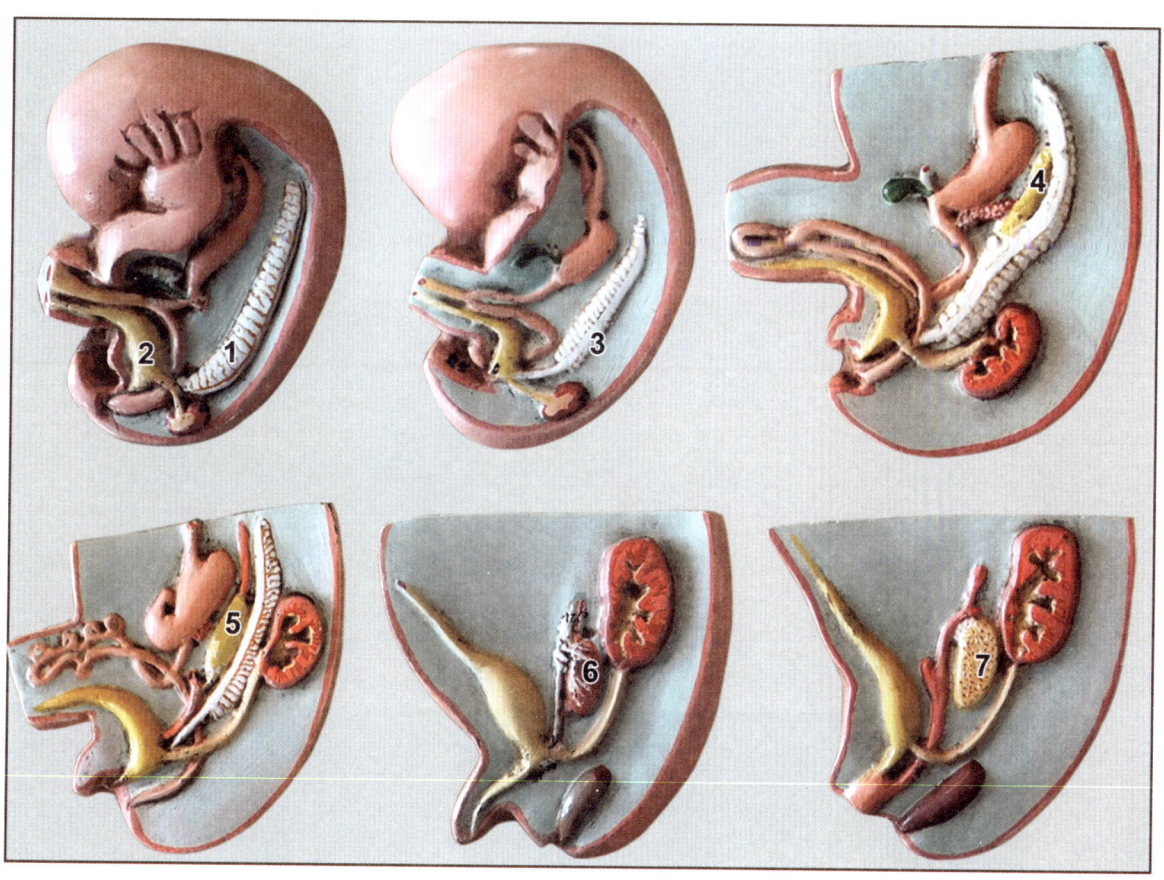

1. ....
2. ....
3. ....
4. ....
5. ....
6. ....
7. ....

1. Which part of intraembryonic mesoderm gives rise to gonads?

....

....

....

2. What is gonadal ridge?

....

....

....

3. What is indifferent gonad?

....

....

....

4. What are primary sex cords?

....

....

....

5. What are secondary sex cords?

....

....

....

6. What is the source of development of leydig cells and sertoli cells?

....

....

....

42 Development of Female Genital Tract

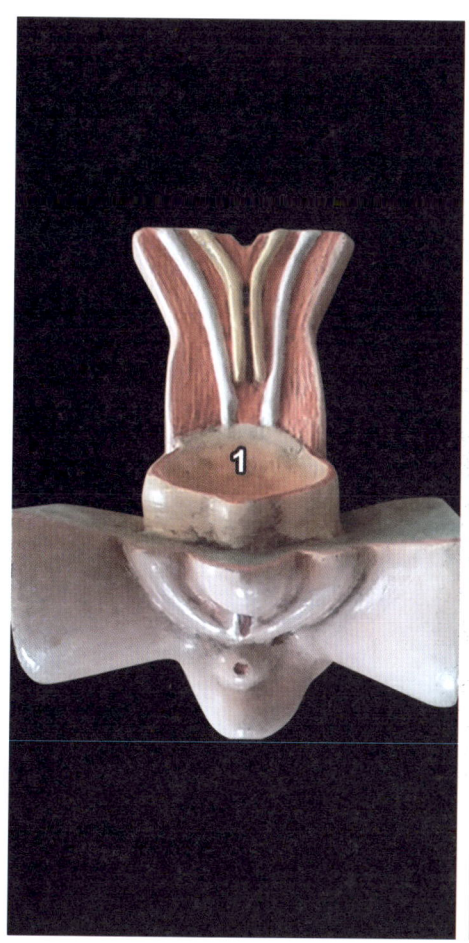 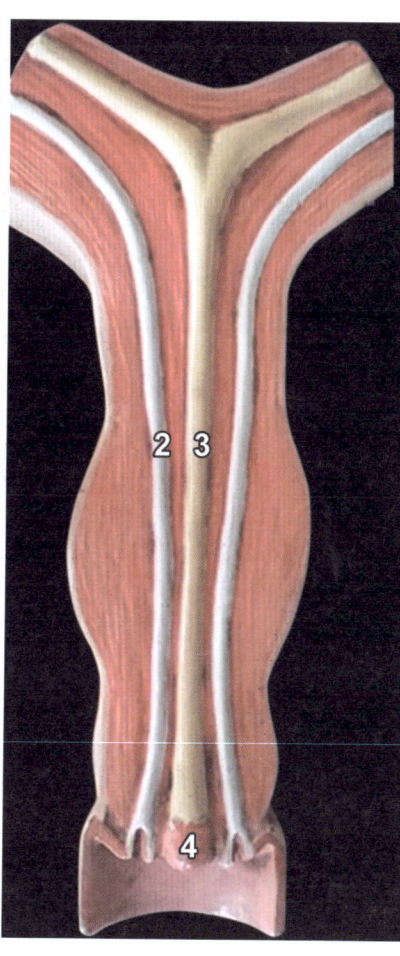 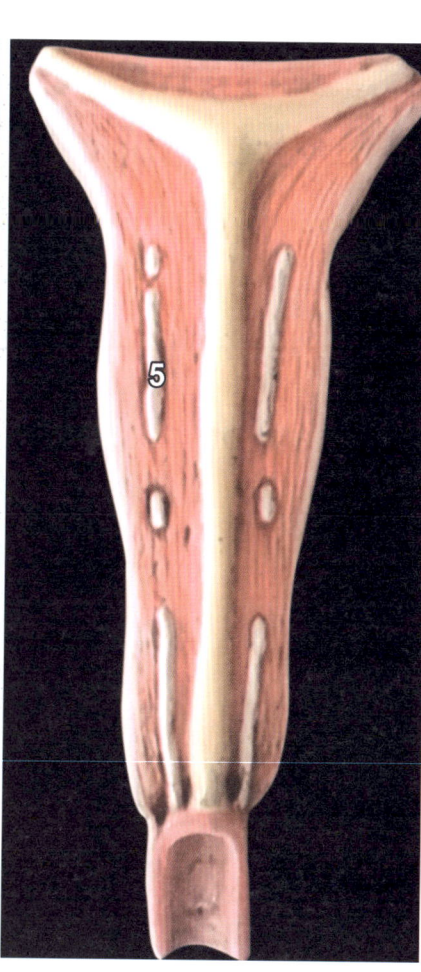

1. ....
2. ....
3. ....
4. ....
5. ....

43

Urogenital Sinus

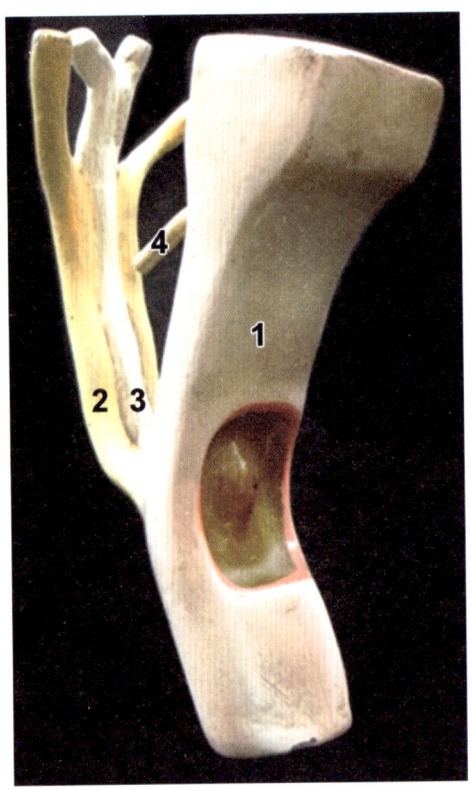

1. ....
2. ....
3. ....
4. ....

1. What are the derivatives of mesonephric duct (wolffian duct) in male?

....

....

....

....

....

2. What are the derivatives of paramesonephric duct (müllerian duct) in females?

....

....

....

....

....

3. Write the remnants of mesonephric duct in females.

....

....

....

....

....

4. Write the remnants of paramesonephric duct in males.

....

....

....

....

....

44

Anomalies of Descent of Testis

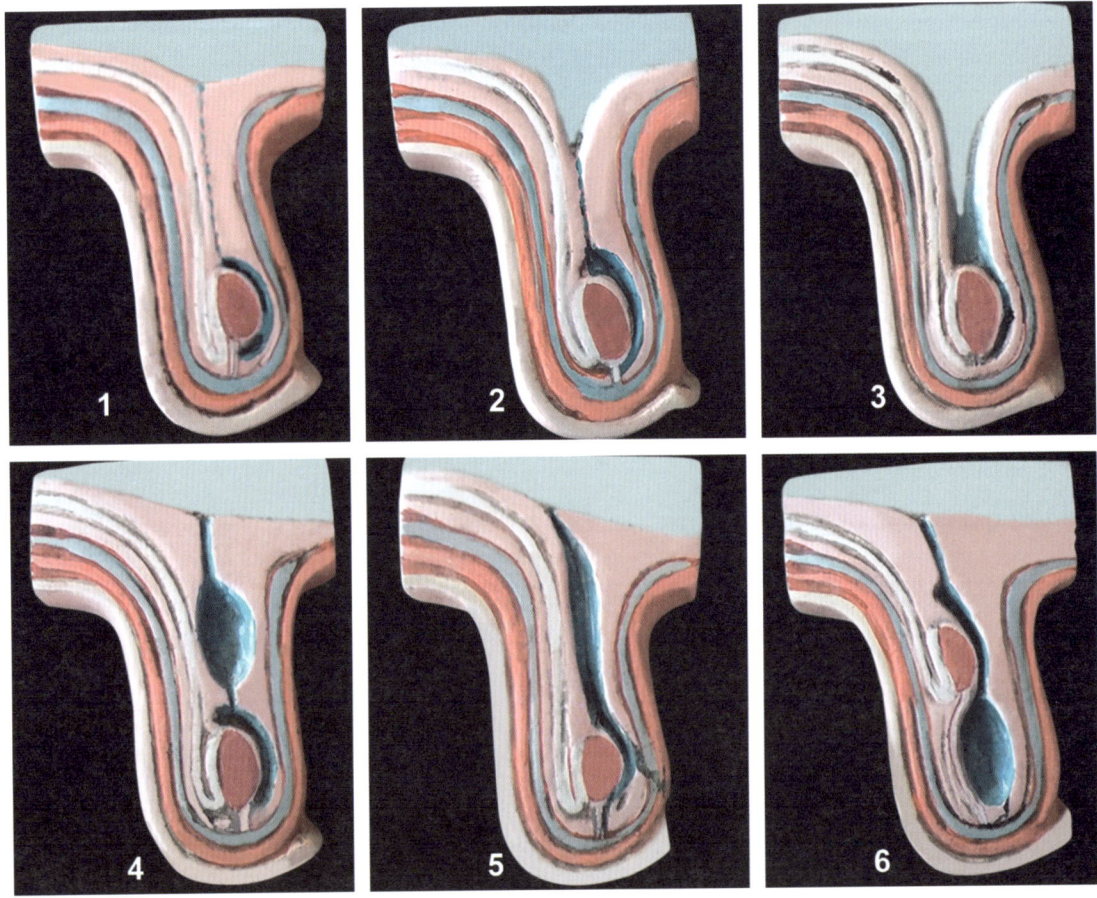

1. ....

2. ....

3. ....

4. ....

5. ....

6. ....

1. What is processus vaginalis?

....

....

....

....

....

....

....

....

2. Explain the process of descent of testis.

....

....

....

....

....

....

....

....

....

3. Mention the factors responsible for descent of testis.

....

....

....

....

....

....

....

....

Anomalies of Uterus

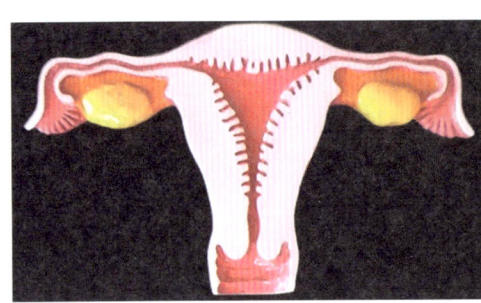

1. ....

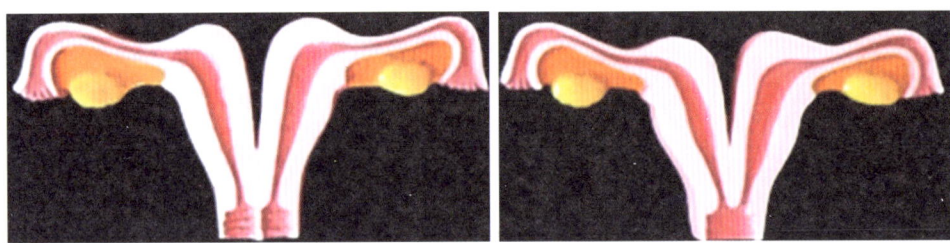

2. .... 3. ....

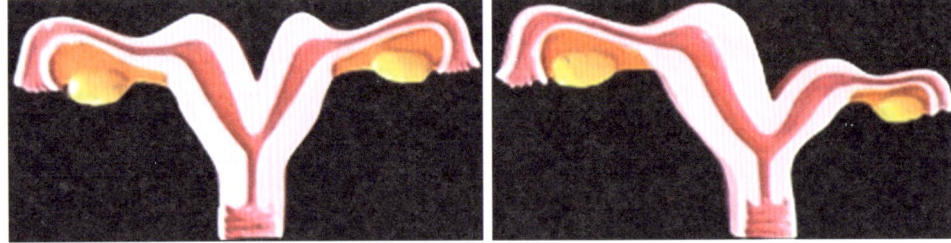

4. .... 5. ....

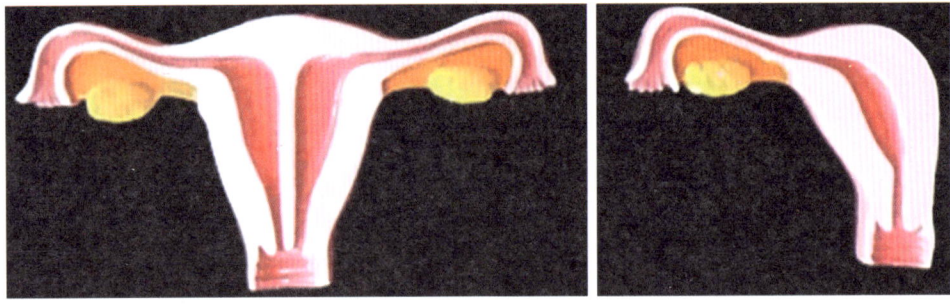

6. .... 7. ....